BARKLEY SLUGGISH COGNITIVE TEMPO SCALE—CHILDREN AND ADOLESCENTS (BSCTS-CA)

Selected Works from Russell A. Barkley

FOR PROFESSIONALS

Attention-Deficit Hyperactivity Disorder, Fourth Edition:
A Handbook for Diagnosis and Treatment
Edited by Russell A. Barkley

Child Psychopathology, Third Edition
Edited by Eric J. Mash and Russell A. Barkley

Defiant Children, Third Edition:
A Clinician's Manual for Assessment and Parent Training
Russell A. Barkley

Defiant Teens, Second Edition:
A Clinician's Manual for Assessment and Family Intervention
Russell A. Barkley and Arthur L. Robin

Executive Functions:
What They Are, How They Work, and Why They Evolved
Russell A. Barkley

FOR GENERAL READERS

Taking Charge of ADHD, Third Edition:
The Complete, Authoritative Guide for Parents
Russell A. Barkley

Your Defiant Child, Second Edition: Eight Steps to Better Behavior
Russell A. Barkley and Christine M. Benton

Your Defiant Teen, Second Edition:
10 Steps to Resolve Conflict and Rebuild Your Relationship
Russell A. Barkley and Arthur L. Robin with Christine M. Benton

ADULT ASSESSMENT SCALES

Barkley Adult ADHD Rating Scale–IV (BAARS-IV)
Russell A. Barkley

Barkley Deficits in Executive Functioning Scale (BDEFS for Adults)
Russell A. Barkley

Barkley Functional Impairment Scale (BFIS for Adults)
Russell A. Barkley

CHILD ASSESSMENT SCALES

Barkley Deficits in Executive Functioning Scale—
Children and Adolescents (BDEFS-CA)
Russell A. Barkley

Barkley Functional Impairment Scale—
Children and Adolescents (BFIS-CA)
Russell A. Barkley

Barkley Sluggish Cognitive Tempo Scale—Children and Adolescents (BSCTS-CA)

Russell A. Barkley

THE GUILFORD PRESS
New York London

For Ken, Heather, and Claire

A Division of Guilford Publications, Inc.
370 Seventh Avenue, Suite 1200, New York, NY 10001
www.guilford.com

Printed in the United States of America

This book is printed on acid-free paper.

Last digit is print number: 9 8 7 6 5 4 3 2 1

Library of Congress Cataloging-in-Publication Data

Names: Barkley, Russell A., 1949– author.
Title: Barkley sluggish cognitive tempo scale—children and adolescents (BSCTS-CA) / Russell Barkley.
Description: New York, NY : The Guilford Press, [2018] | Includes bibliographical references and index.
Identifiers: LCCN 2018001059 | ISBN 9781462535187 (pbk. : alk. paper)
Subjects: | MESH: Attention Deficit and Disruptive Behavior Disorders—diagnosis | Cognition Disorders—diagnosis | Child | Adolescent
Classification: LCC RJ506.C63 | NLM WS 350.6 | DDC 618.92/89—dc23
LC record available at https://lccn.loc.gov/2018001059

About the Author

Russell A. Barkley, PhD, ABPP, ABCN, is Clinical Professor of Psychiatry at the Virginia Treatment Center for Children and Virginia Commonwealth University School of Medicine. Dr. Barkley has worked with children, adolescents, and families since the 1970s and is the author of numerous bestselling books for both professionals and the public, including *Taking Charge of ADHD* and *Your Defiant Child.* He has also published six assessment scales and more than 280 scientific articles and book chapters on ADHD, executive functioning, and childhood defiance, and is editor of the newsletter *The ADHD Report.* A frequent conference presenter and speaker who is widely cited in the national media, Dr. Barkley is past president of the Section on Clinical Child Psychology (the former Division 12) of the American Psychological Association (APA), and of the International Society for Research in Child and Adolescent Psychopathology. He is a recipient of awards from the American Academy of Pediatrics and the APA, among other honors. His website is *www.russellbarkley.org.*

Acknowledgments

This manual describes the development, validation, and norming of a parent's version of the Barkley Sluggish Cognitive Tempo Scale—Children and Adolescents (BSCTS-CA) that can be used in the evaluation of both attention-deficit/hyperactivity disorder and sluggish cognitive tempo in children, also known as concentration deficit disorder. I wish to thank Wendy Mansfield and Sergei Rodkin of Knowledge Networks (Menlo Park, California) for their assistance with the collection of the normative sample of parents used to create the norms for the BSCTS-CA in this manual. I sincerely appreciate the assistance of Anna Brackett of The Guilford Press for her expert production editing of this manual. I continue to express my deep appreciation to Kitty Moore, Seymour Weingarten, and Bob Matloff at Guilford for their acceptance, support of, and assistance with this normative project and the publication of the BSCTS-CA.

Contents

Introduction

This manual reports on the history, normative data, psychometric properties, and scoring and interpretation for the Barkley Sluggish Cognitive Tempo Scale—Children and Adolescents (BSCTS-CA) and its clinical use for children ages 6–17 years. The Appendix to this manual contains the rating scale of the BSCTS-CA for parents. There is also a parent interview version based on the rating scale for use in unusual circumstances in which a parent is unable to complete a rating scale. Profiles are also provided for converting the raw scores from the rating scale to percentiles for the child's age group (6–11 years or 12–17 years) and sex.

The BSCTS-CA is the culmination of more than 10 years of research and development on identifying the most useful items for the assessment of concentration deficits or symptoms of sluggish cognitive tempo (SCT) in the daily life activities of children and teens, as observed by their parents. The BSCTS-CA is *empirically developed,* based on statistical analyses that were used to identify the most reliable and valid symptoms of concentration problems and their underlying dimensions in daily life. Not only is the BSCTS-CA empirically based, it is also quite reliable and has numerous lines of evidence of its validity, as established here and in the scientific literature. It is also exceptionally convenient to use, due largely to the willingness of the publisher to grant the purchasers of this manual a limited permission to photocopy the scales and score sheets for use in their clinical practice or research projects. This benefit saves the purchaser a great deal of time, inconvenience, and expense typically associated with the continual reordering of those scales and scoring sheets, as is commonplace in the scale publishing industry.

This manual begins with a brief introduction to the concept of SCT in clinical psychology and its differentiation from another attention disorder, attention-deficit/hyperactivity disorder (ADHD). I then provide details of the developmental history of the initial BSCTS-CA and its progression to this parent report form. The remaining chapters provide information on the normative sample, factor analysis, and other information concerning the scale's reliability, validity, and clinical utility, along with instructions for scoring and interpretation of the scale. The information available appears to be sufficient to recommend the use of the scale in a variety of circumstances. These may include clinical practice settings with parents of children who are concerned about possible concentration deficits in the child or teen beyond those inattention symptoms sampled by traditional ADHD rating scales; in research settings where the evaluation of SCT symptoms relative to those of ADHD in children and teens is a specific aim; in treatment trials as a measure of response to child- and parent-focused interventions in which a child's SCT or ADHD symptoms are of interest; or in school settings where the screening of children for possible concentration deficits inherent in SCT or ADHD, as reported by their parents, is an important objective. I hope you will find the BSCTS-CA rating scales to be useful in the evaluation of both ADHD and SCT symptoms in children and teens in their daily life activities, as reported by their parents.

CHAPTER 1

A Review of Research on SCT

This introductory chapter briefly reviews the evidence supporting the conclusion that a second attention disorder exists, known as "sluggish cognitive tempo" (SCT), which is distinct from, yet overlaps with, ADHD. The review is adapted from my earlier chapter on this topic (Barkley, 2015a) but updated with the numerous research studies and a meta-analysis that were published thereafter. The abbreviation "SCT" has been in use since the term was first coined in the 1980s, based on research studying dimensions of attention problems in children with ADHD. Along with other researchers, I believe the term "sluggish cognitive tempo" is far from ideal, and many are recommending it be changed to something less derogatory, pejorative, or, frankly, offensive. I have suggested that the name be changed to concentration deficit disorder (CDD) for this precise reason (Barkley, 2014; Saxbe & Barkley, 2014).

Some prior reviews have suggested that the condition be called "attention-deficit disorder" (ADD; Diamond, 2005). Many clinicians have adopted this term for people who are primarily inattentive and have little or no evidence of hyperactive or impulsive behavior. Although some of those cases likely involve SCT, I do not believe it is advisable to use the term "ADD" for this heterogeneous group. For one reason, ADD is the older term for ADHD, dating back to the third edition of the *Diagnostic and Statistical Manual of Mental Disorders* (DSM-III; American Psychiatric Association, 1980). Resurrecting ADD as the name for a second attention disorder that is distinct in many ways from ADHD serves to create unnecessary confusion between the conditions. Moreover, ADD could be inferred to be a type or presentation of ADHD, such as is the primarily inattentive presentation now set forth in DSM-5 (American Psychiatric Association, 2013). As for continuing to use the term "SCT," the name clearly implies that the core cognitive deficit(s) underlying the condition has been definitively established (slow timing of thinking or information processing), which is not true. The same criticism can be applied to other terms suggested for something similar to this condition, such as primary disorder of vigilance (PDV; Weinberg & Brumback, 1990, 1992; Weinberg & Harper, 1993).

CDD, I believe, seems to be a reasonable option as an alternative label for SCT for various reasons: (1) It has not been used for any other disorder previously; (2) it keeps the focus of the label on an attention problem yet makes it distinct from ADHD; (3) it is not offensive or pejorative to patients and family members, as is SCT; (4) it does not imply that we know more than we do about the underlying cognitive dysfunction, as do SCT and PDV; and (5) it suggests some overlap with ADHD, which is the case (see Barkley, 2014). Moreover, the term "concentration" does not appear in the symptom lists for either ADHD (DSM-5) or SCT (Penny, Waschbusch, Klein, Corkum, & Eskes, 2009) and thus is less likely to create unnecessary semantic confusion. Throughout the remainder of this chapter, I refer to this condition as SCT, because it is a review of the history and findings related to that condition, in contrast to what is seen in ADHD. I wish to remain true to the term as used by other researchers in discussing their own findings, at least for the time being, until the field can reach some consensus on a less derogatory term.

History of SCT versus ADHD

Cases of SCT have likely existed within the human population at least throughout the past two centuries, if not longer. Descriptions of individuals with "low power" of attention or arousal, who appear to stare or daydream frequently, and who otherwise seem inattentive or sluggish and erratic in accurately processing information seem to first appear in the literature in Crichton's medical textbook, wherein he provided us with a description of two disorders of attention (Crichton, 1798/1976; also see Palmer & Finger, 2001). One disorder clearly resembles what today we label as ADHD. In contrast to it, Crichton had little to say about the other disorder of attention, except that it may be associated with debility or torpor of the body that weakens attention, thus causing individuals to be retiring, unsocial, and to have few friends or attachments of any kind. SCT may also have been the subject of a nursery rhyme written by the German psychiatrist Heinrich Hoffman, entitled "Johnny Head-in-the-Air," which was contained in his illustrated children's storybook, *Der Struwwelpeter,* published in 1865. The book is often cited as an early reference to ADHD, as represented in "The Story of Fidgety Philip."

Apart from such historical curiosities, the contemporary period of research on SCT began in the 1980s and was clearly a consequence of the creation of two types of ADD in DSM-III (American Psychiatric Association, 1980): ADD with (+H) and without (–H) hyperactivity. Studies soon began to appear that examined differences between children having each type of ADD (Carlson, 1986; Lahey, Schaughency, Strauss, & Frame, 1984; Maurer & Stewart, 1980; Milich, Ballentine, & Lynam, 2001). Their findings met with mixed success in differentiating the two types on features other than what would have been evident from their symptom requirements. That led to the removal of this subtyping approach in the subsequent DSM-III-R (American Psychiatric Association, 1987), only to see it return in the subtyping framework contained in DSM-IV as ADHD, combined type, versus ADHD, predominantly inattentive type (American Psychiatric Association, 1994). This subtyping method was demoted again to the status of a mere "presentation" in the most recent DSM (DSM-5; American Psychiatric Association, 2013).

The specific identification of SCT seems to have begun in 1984 when Lahey and colleagues (1984) compared just 10 children with ADD+H to 20 children with ADD–H. They reported that the ADD+H group had significantly higher levels of aggressive behavior and conduct problems, bizarre behavior, lack of guilt, peer unpopularity, and poor performance in school. In comparison, the ADD–H children were more likely to be anxious, shy, socially withdrawn, and moderately unpopular, as well as poor in sports and impaired in school performance, all of which would later be replicated as correlates of SCT. The authors identified a set of symptoms in the ADD–H group that seemed to best characterize their attention problems but that were not part of the DSM symptom lists. Those symptoms included drowsiness, sluggishness, and daydreaming, among others (Carlson, personal communication, November 20, 2013). In 1985, according to Carlson (1986), a student of Lahey's (Neeper) conducted a cluster analysis in order to subtype learning-disabled children on the basis of their behavior by using a rating scale that contained these and other items (see also Carlson, Lahey, & Neeper, 1986). He identified a separate group of 11 children having high scores on an inattention–disorganization factor and low scores in motor hyperactivity. That separate factor was then named a "sluggish tempo factor" and comprised items related to apathetic, lethargic, sluggish, and drowsy behaviors. The condition has been referred to as "sluggish cognitive tempo" ever since.

In 2001, a very influential review of the literature concerning the two attention disorders (ADD+H and ADD–H) was published by Milich and colleagues (2001). The authors comprehensively reviewed research regarding comparisons of the subtypes. They also reviewed research using factor analysis of ratings of inattention. That research identified three distinct factors, two of which characterized ADHD: inattention and hyperactive–impulsive symptoms. SCT symptoms formed a third and distinct factor from these other two dimensions, and so the label SCT was applied to it. This was also found to be the case in a factor analysis of the direct observation form of the Child Behavior Checklist by McConaughy and Achenbach (2001), in which a separate attention deficit emerged independent of that typifying ADHD. Also in 2001, McBurnett et al. conducted a factor analysis of ratings collected on 692 children referred to a specialty pediatric clinic for ADHD and found, as did Neeper earlier (dissertation research cited in Carlson et al., 1986), that symptoms labeled as SCT formed a distinct dimension from the two traditional ones comprising ADHD. Three years later, Todd and colleagues (Todd, Rasmussen, Wood, Levy, & Hay, 2004) factor-analyzed data from 2,894 twin pairs and also found a separate factor for SCT symptoms distinct from those for ADHD. Such a factor would emerge from all subsequent studies of the symptom lists of ADHD and SCT.

In the past decade, studies have focused specifically on children identified with high levels of SCT symptoms, in comparison to those with ADHD. Some studies have estimated that as many as 30–63% of cases of the predominantly inattentive cases of ADHD have high levels of SCT (Carlson & Mann, 2002; Garner et al., 2010; McBurnett et al., 2001). Subsequently, many researchers have focused on groups of children, and later adults, with high levels of SCT symptoms (Barkley, 2012a,

2013; Carlson & Mann, 2002; Garner, Marceaux, Mrug, Patterson, & Hodgens, 2010; McBurnett et al., 2001; Penny et al., 2009; Skirbekk, Hansen, Oerbeck, & Kristensen, 2011). Indeed, Penny et al. went so far as to compile a comprehensive set of SCT symptoms based on answers from experts they surveyed and their review of research papers. They then subjected the items to further analysis, ultimately creating a rating scale of the most useful set. By 2012, I had developed the first SCT rating scale for adults and published the results of the first study of adult SCT based on a representative U.S. sample of adults ages 18–92 (Barkley, 2012a), discussed further below. At the same time, I created a 12-item rating scale of SCT symptoms for children that was given to a representative sample of 1,922 U.S. parents to complete (Barkley, 2013) and that serves as the basis for this manual and the BSCTS-CA.

In summation, the construct of SCT grew out of efforts to identify differences between subtypes of ADD and subsequently children with ADHD. Whereas differences between those subtypes proved mixed, weak, and unconvincing of any substantial or qualitative differences (Willcutt et al., 2012), research focusing specifically on children (and later, adults) having high levels of SCT symptoms proved much more promising in consistently identifying a variety of distinctions from ADHD. By 2016, sufficient research on SCT made it possible to conduct a meta-analysis of the existing literature, which would conclude that on a number of variables, SCT seemed to be distinct from ADHD and worthy of much further study (Becker et al., 2016). Even so, in comparison to ADHD, the condition of SCT remains a highly understudied problem with fewer than 70 articles currently existing on SCT in children and perhaps no more than 20 on adults (Becker, Burns, Garner, et al., 2017). Increased demand for such empirically based knowledge is likely to appear due to increasing clinical referrals of cases with this condition, driven by the general public's increased awareness of SCT. The fact that SCT does not yet exist in any official taxonomy of psychiatric disorders does not alter this prediction. The increasing information on SCT at various widely visited Internet sites such as YouTube and Wikipedia, among others, will ensure a growing public demand for more scientific knowledge about SCT and its management.

What Do We Know about the Nature of SCT Compared to ADHD?

The Best Symptoms for Identifying SCT

Although there is no official symptom list for SCT, as there is for ADHD, researchers have identified its most salient symptoms (Barkley, 2012a, 2013; Becker, Leopold, et al., 2016; Becker, Burns, Garner, et al., 2017; Garner et al., 2010; McBurnett et al., 2001; Penny et al., 2009). My own research found the best symptoms for identifying SCT to be the following (Barkley, 2013): (1) daydreaming; (2) trouble staying awake/alert; (3) feeling mentally foggy/easily confused; (4) staring a lot; (5) looks/feel spacey, mind is elsewhere; (6) is lethargic; (7) is underactive; (8) is slow-moving/sluggish; (9) doesn't process questions or explanations accurately; (10) appears drowsy/sleepy; (11) appears apathetic/withdrawn; (12) is lost in thoughts; (13) slow to complete tasks; and (14) lacks initiative/effort fades. The last two symptoms, however, were as likely to be associated with ADHD as with SCT in children and adolescents. Therefore, they are not recommended for assisting with differential diagnosis between these two types of attention disorders (Barkley, 2013; Burns, Servera, Bernad, Carrillo, & Cardo, 2013; Lee, Burns, Snell, & McBurnett, 2013) and do not appear in the BSCTS-CA contained in this manual. But the remaining 12, among others (Becker, Burns, Garner, et al., 2017; Penny et al., 2009), are highly useful for identifying cases of SCT and so were used to form the BSCTS-CA in this manual.

Recently, the meta-analysis by Becker, Leopold, and colleagues (2016) identified a set of 13 symptoms that seemed most useful to identifying SCT, primarily in children, given that most such research in that analysis used that population. Subsequently, Becker, Burns, Garner, et al. (2017) developed a rating scale of SCT symptoms for adults, in which they studied 16 symptoms for potential use in their Adult Concentration Inventory (ACI). As is shown in Table 1.1, most of the symptoms from the meta-analysis are contained in their ACI scale. And the validation study in adults found that 10 of those symptoms on the ACI were most useful for identifying SCT in adults (distinguishing it from ADHD). Table 1.1 shows the results of these two efforts to identify the best candidate symptoms.

It should be noted that 10 of the 13 best items identified in the meta-analysis are contained on the BSCTS-CA form, and 8 of the 10 items from the adult validation

TABLE 1.1. ACI Items and Support from Meta-Analysis and Validation in Adults

ACI items	SCT meta-analysis	Validation in adults
1. I am slow at doing things.	✓	×
2. My mind feels like it is in a fog.	✓	×
3. I stare off into space.	✓	✓
4. I feel sleepy or drowsy during the day.	✓	✓
5. I lose my train of thought.	✓	✓
6. I am not very active.	✓	×
7. I get lost in my own thoughts.	✓	✓
8. I get tired easily.	✓	✓
9. I forget what I was going to say.	×	✓
10. I feel confused.	✓	✓
11. I am not motivated to do things.	✓	×
12. I zone out or space out.	✓	✓
13. My mind gets mixed up.	×	✓
14. My thinking seems slow or slowed down	✓	×
15. I daydream	✓	✓
16. I have a hard time putting my thoughts	×	×

Note. The meta-analysis is from Becker, Leopold, et al. (2016), and the adult validation study is from Becker, Burns, Garner, et al. (2017).

study likewise appear on this form. Note should be made here that symptom 11 was found in earlier research to be as much associated with ADHD as with SCT, and so was not a useful item, at least for children (discussed above). And symptoms 5, 7, 9, 13, and 16, or items similar to them, were found in factor analyses of the national survey reported later in this manual to be far more strongly associated with a dimension of executive functioning (EF) in daily life related to self-organization (Barkley Deficits in Executive Functioning Scale—Children and Adolescents [BDEFS-CA; Barkley, 2012d]) and not to SCT. So 6 of the 16 items from the meta-analysis noted in Table 1.1 should not really be used to identify SCT because they will likely contaminate the construct with either ADHD (in the case of item 11) or EF (in the case of items 5, 7, 9, 13, and 16). This is why they are not contained on the BSCTS-CA in this manual.

More recently, Becker and colleagues (Becker, Burns, Schmitt, Epstein, & Tamm, 2017) conducted a large study of 1,349 children in grades 2–5 using the following 16 items:

1. Behavior is slow (e.g., sluggish) (0.92)
2. Lost in a fog (0.89)
3. Stares blankly into space (0.96)
4. Drowsy or sleepy (yawns) during the day (0.95)
5. Daydreams (0.88)
6. Loses train of thought (0.86)
7. Low level of activity (e.g., underactive) (0.97)
8. Gets lost in own thoughts (0.81)
9. Easily tired or fatigued (1.02)
10. Forgets what was going to say (0.94)
11. Easily confused (0.91)
12. Lacks motivation to complete tasks (e.g., apathetic) (0.27)
13. Spaces or zones out (0.82)
14. Gets mixed up (0.85)
15. Thinking is slow (0.87)
16. Difficulty expressing thoughts (e.g., gets "tongue-tied") (0.78)

In their exploratory and confirmatory factor analysis (contrasting these items with those of ADHD inattention), Becker, Burns, Garner, et al. (2017) found that 15 of these 16 symptoms loaded highly on an SCT factor (factor loadings are in parentheses beside each symptom) and not significantly on the ADHD inattention factor. Item 12 did not, however; it was far more highly linked to the ADHD inattention symptom dimension. As noted previously, this finding again corroborates earlier research that this item dealing with motivation is not a good symptom for identifying SCT from ADHD.

Of the remaining 15 symptoms, the authors found that item 14 (Gets mixed up) was highly correlated and thus redundant with item 11 (Easily confused) and so is unnecessary to include in a symptom list. And items 6, 10, and 16, dealing with problems organizing and expressing thoughts, were found to be most highly associated with that dimension of EF in daily life related to self-organization, not to SCT, in the factor analysis to be reported later. The Becker, Burns, Schmitt, et al. (2017) study did not use any measures of EF in daily life, and so these three items appeared to load instead on their SCT dimension. As discussed below, prior research has shown that SCT has a small but significant association with this dimension of EF, so it is not surprising that in the absence of any EF measures, these items would seem to align with SCT. Yet given the opportunity to be analyzed alongside other EF symptoms, these apparent SCT symptoms then migrate over to the self-organization dimension of EF and do not remain useful SCT items. For this reason, I again do not believe they should appear on a list of the best items for identifying SCT.

With these issues in mind, that leaves just 11 of the 16 items on the preceding list as representing the best symptoms for identifying SCT. All 11 of these symptoms appear on the BSCTS-CA, though not necessarily worded exactly as they appear here. Also, two (2 and 11) of the symptoms on the preceding list are contained in a single item on the BSCTS-CA (Mentally foggy or easily confused). And the BSCTS-CA has an extra symptom reflecting difficulties remaining alert or awake that does not appear on the Becker, Burns, Schmitt, et al. list. Item 15 (Thinking is slow) is represented on the BSCTS-CA as "Doesn't seem to understand or process questions or explanations as quickly or accurately as others." More on the phrasing and derivation of the SCT symptoms on the BSCTS-CA is presented in subsequent chapters, including the results of my factor analysis in comparison to ADHD and EF symptoms.

Thus, for now, it is safe to say that the BSCTS-CA utilizes the vast majority, if not all, of the best symptoms identified in prior research as optimal for differentiating SCT from ADHD, as well as other disorders and EF, even though it was initially developed prior to these two research reports by Becker and colleagues.

The Symptom Dimensions Are Distinct from ADHD

In prior research the symptoms of SCT seem to form either a single factor (Becker, Burns, Schmitt, et al., 2017) or at least two factors or dimensions. Those two identified dimensions are intercorrelated sufficiently to be combined in identifying this disorder. Most commonly, the two dimensions identified in factor-analytic research are a Daydreamy/Spacey factor and a Sleepy/Sluggish/Underactive dimension or factor (Barkley, 2013; Burns et al., 2013; Jacobson et al., 2012; Mueller et al., 2014; Penny et al., 2009). In a study of adolescents with ADHD, a Sleepy dimension emerged that was somewhat distinct from the Daydreamy and Sluggish factors (Smith & Langberg, 2017), but this is not the case in studies of children or when child and teenage samples are combined (Barkley, 2013). In some studies, a separate factor is found for the low initiative and lack of persistence items (see 13 and 14 above). But as noted, these two seem to be more related to ADHD inattentive symptoms than to SCT and thus would not be useful in differentiating SCT from ADHD (Barkley, 2013). Interestingly, as with ADHD, there is a cognitive-inattentive dimension (Daydreamy/Spacey) and a motor dimension (Sluggish/Lethargic) to SCT, though they are clearly different from the symptoms comprising those general dimensions in ADHD. Smith and Langberg (2017) have argued that, at least in adolescents with ADHD, a multidimensional view of SCT, as discussed previously, is preferable to a unidimensional view, given that the different dimensions appear to predict different forms of impairment (academic vs. internalizing problems).

The distinctiveness of SCT and its factors from those of ADHD have been evident across all of the various approaches to measurement studied to date, such as parent and teacher ratings (Barkley, 2013; Bauermeister, Barkley, Bauermeister, Martinez, & McBurnett, 2012; Becker, Burns, Schmitt, et al., 2017; Becker, Luebbe, Fite, Stoppelbein, & Greening, 2014; Burns et al., 2013; Garner et al., 2010; Hartman, Willcutt, Rhee, & Pennington, 2004; Jacobson et al., 2012; Lee et al., 2013; McBurnett, Villodas, Burns, Hinshaw, Beaulieu, & Pfiffner, 2014; Penny et al., 2009; Willcutt et al., 2013), observations of behavior at school (McConaughy, Ivanova, Antshel, Eiraldi, & Dumenci, 2009), and observations of behavior in clinical settings (McConaughy, Ivanova, Antshel, & Eiraldi, 2009). SCT symptoms are distinct not only from those of children with ADHD (Barkley, 2013) and youth (Smith & Langberg, 2017), but are also found to be distinct from those of adults with ADHD in self-reports for ages 18–89 years (Barkley, 2012a) and among college students (Becker, Burns, Garner, et al., 2017).

Despite finding SCT symptoms to be distinct from those of ADHD across ages, measures, and even sources, they may not necessarily correlate strongly across measurement sources. For instance, several studies have found only a low-to-moderate relationship between parent and teacher rated symptoms (*r*s = .29–.38; Koriakin, Mahone, & Jacobson, 2015; Markovich-Pilon, Corkum, & Joyce, 2017), showing that at most, these ratings share just 14% of their variance. Although disappointing, such correlations are in keeping with the usual and modest levels of association found between parent and teacher ratings of all dimensions of child psychopathology (Achenbach, McConaughy, & Howell, 1987).

SCT Symptoms Are Moderately Related to ADHD Inattention but Not to Hyperactivity–Impulsivity

SCT symptoms have been found repeatedly to be significantly but moderately correlated with the ADHD inattention symptom dimension, suggesting about 25–36% shared variance between the two dimensions. Hence, they are not identical, nor do they approach colinearity as if they derived from the same item pool or construct. Moreover, SCT symptoms identify a unique group of children even within samples that include ADHD inattentive type (Capdivila-Brophy et al., 2012; Marshall, Evans, Eiraldi, Becker, & Power, 2013). Yet SCT symptoms are substantially less correlated with ADHD symptoms than they are with each other (Barkley, 2012a, 2013; Penney et al., 2009). A number of studies find that SCT symptoms demonstrate a much weaker relationship to hyperactive–impulsive symptoms, if at all, than they do to inattention symptoms (Barkley, 2012a, 2012b; Burns et al., 2013; Hartman et al., 2004; Garner et al., 2010; Jacobson et al., 2012; Penny et al., 2009; Wahlstedt & Bohlin, 2010). In fact, this relationship may become negative, at least for the SCT slowness dimension, once ADHD inattention is statistically removed (Lee et al., 2013; Penny et al., 2009). All of this is to say that the structure of SCT symptoms is not merely a reflection or broadening of the ADHD inattention symptom dimension.

Instead, SCT symptoms are as independent or as only partially coupled to ADHD symptoms as are other symptom dimensions of child and adult psychopathology to each other.

SCT Symptoms Are Evident and Valid in Other Cultures/Countries

A small but growing body of evidence indicates that SCT symptoms can be identified in samples from other countries and cultures, and that they show a similar pattern of distinctiveness from ADHD symptoms. Thus there is cross-cultural validity to this condition, at least as examined to date. Studies using samples of children from *Canada* (Markovich-Pilon et al., 2017), *Spain* (Burns et al., 2013; Camprodon-Rosanas et al., 2017a; Camprodon-Rosanas et al., 2017b; Preszler et al., 2017), *Korea* (Lee, Burns, & Becker, 2016), *Nepal* (Khada, Burns, & Becker, 2016), and *Chile* (Belmar, Servera, Becker, & Burns, 2015) all attest to the existence and validity of SCT within these countries as a distinct condition from ADHD, so it is not strictly a U.S. phenomenon. This cross-cultural existence and validity are true of ADHD as well.

In sum, individual studies and meta-analyses of symptoms of SCT show that they:

- Are coherent among themselves (more highly correlated with each other than with symptoms of other disorders, e.g., ADHD).
- Form a distinct dimension or set of dimensions of symptoms from those comprising other disorders, such as ADHD, anxiety, and depression.
- Are internally consistent (high internal reliability).
- Show reasonable test–retest reliability over short time periods (Becker et al., 2016).
- Have significant stability and invariance over long periods, from 2 (Servera, Bernad, Carillo, Collado, & Burns, 2016) to 9 years (Leopold et al., 2016).
- Show comparable low-to-moderate relationships between parent and teacher ratings, as seen in other child psychopathologies.
- Are evident cross-culturally.

Demographic Differences in SCT and ADHD

Relationships to Age and Sex

Only a handful of prior studies examined parental/family demographic characteristics of SCT versus ADHD. Several studies (Garner et al., 2010; Jacobson et al., 2012) found that SCT was not related to child age, gender, or minority status. This same pattern was evident in my two large epidemiological studies of representative samples of U.S. children (Barkley, 2013) and adults (Barkley, 2012a) across ages 6–89 years. This was also the conclusion of the meta-analysis by Becker, Leopold, Burns, and colleagues (2016), in which only a slight relationship of SCT symptoms to age was noted. In ADHD, however, the symptoms decline with age across childhood, especially those of hyperactive–impulsive symptoms. Groups having SCT have also been noted to be older than those having ADHD (Becker, Leopold, Burns, et al., 2016), implying a somewhat later age of onset for the former symptoms.

Boys demonstrated more ADHD symptoms than girls during childhood and adolescence but come close to being nearly equal in adulthood (Barkley, 2012a, 2013; Burns et al., 2013). This is not the case for SCT: Males have only a slightly greater number of symptoms than females in childhood and no evident sex differences in symptom occurrence by adulthood (Barkley, 2012a, 2013; Becker, Burns, Schmitt, et al., 2017; Burns et al., 2013). This lack of, or very small association of, SCT with age and sex was also evident in a study by Lee et al. (2013), who noted no sex differences and no effect of age on teacher ratings and only a very small difference due to those demographic factors in parent ratings.

Some studies have found ADHD symptoms to be slightly but statistically significantly associated with some ethnic groups (e.g., Hispanic/Latino) more than others, whereas this is not the case for SCT symptoms, either in large nationally representative samples (Barkley, 2012a, 2013) or in the meta-analysis by Becker, Leopold, and colleagues (2016).

Relations with Parental Factors

In my national survey of children (Barkley, 2013), I noted that SCT was linked to lower parental education, lower annual household income, and a greater likelihood of a parent being out of work due to disability. A study in Spain also noted an association of this symptom dimension with paternal unemployment and low maternal education in a large sample of Catalan school children (Camprodon-Rosanas et al., 2017b). My survey of U.S. adults (Barkley, 2012a) similarly found that those classified as SCT had less education and less annual income. In those instances where SCT was comorbid with ADHD in the adult survey (Barkley, 2012a), those individuals were more likely to be unmarried and out of work on disability than were adults with ADHD. Such findings intimate that SCT might be more associated with psychosocial adversity or stressors than is ADHD. But the meta-analysis by Becker, Leopold, and colleagues (2016) concluded that SCT might be less related to such parental demographic features than ADHD. To summarize, what patterns emerge in results to date indicate that the demographic correlates associated with SCT may be different from, or far weaker than, those evident in ADHD.

Differences in Psychometrically Assessed Cognitive Functioning

In general, there has been vastly less research on the neuropsychological deficits associated with SCT compared to ADHD, where the research literature is abundant (Frazier, Demaree, & Youngstrom, 2004; Hervey, Epstein, & Curry, 2004; Willcutt, Doyle, Nigg, Faraone, & Pennington, 2005; Willcutt, 2015). Studies are not consistent in showing a relationship of SCT to lower levels of intelligence. But the bulk of the evidence suggests a significant but modest negative relationship (Becker, Leopold, et al., 2016) that may be most evident when teacher-rated SCT is the source rather than parent ratings (Markovich-Pilon et al., 2017).

A few studies imply that SCT may involve deficits in early information processing or selective attention that is not typical of ADHD (Huang-Pollack, Nigg, & Carr,

2005). One recent study suggests that preschoolers with high SCT ratings may be more impaired on tests of visual–perceptual abilities, auditory and visual attention, sustained and selective attention, inhibitory control, and prenumerical/numerical concepts, even after controlling for ADHD inattention (Tamm, Brenner, Bamberger, & Becker, 2018). Variability of spatial memory performance has also been specifically linked to SCT but not to ADHD in the Skirbekk et al. (2011) study, even after controlling for IQ, ADHD inattention, and other variables. But such findings from so few studies must be replicated in more research before being viewed as confirmed correlates of SCT.

Likewise, slower processing or motor speed has been linked to hypoactivity specifically (Lundervold, Posserud, Ullebo, Sorensen, & Gillberg, 2011) and to SCT symptoms more generally in some studies of children (Adams, Milich, & Fillmore, 2010; Camprodon-Rosanas et al., 2017a; Garner et al., 2010; Jacobson, Geist, & Mahone, 2017), consistent with SCT's symptom profile. One recent study (Camprodon-Rosanas et al., 2017a) found that teacher-rated SCT symptoms were significantly though modestly correlated with poorer performance on both a working memory (WM) task and the response parameter scores (mean reaction time, reaction time variability) of the attention network task (ANT) with *r*s = –.17–.20 for WM and .20–.22 for ANT. But there was no association of SCT with those scores on the ANT linked to different attention networks (Alerting, Orienting, Conflict). And only the relationship of SCT to slow mean reaction time on the ANT remained significant after controlling for potential confounding variables, including ADHD inattention. In contrast, on reaction time tasks ADHD is repeatedly associated with greater variability of reaction times (Frazier et al., 2004; Hervey et al., 2004; Willcutt et al., 2005).

One question raised by such findings is whether this problem of slow or sluggish speed in responding is the result of difficulties on the information-processing side (perceptual speed) or the motor preparatory and execution side, or both (Jacobson et al., 2017). Current research has not been able to address this issue satisfactorily, yet the results of the Camprodon-Rosanas et al. (2017a) study noted previously imply that it may be more of a motor slowing problem. And the problem of speed, wherever it arises, may not be so evident in older children (Jacobson et al., 2017) and perhaps not at all by college age (Wood, Potts, Lewandowski, & Lovett, 2016). However, as several studies found (e.g., Camprodon-Rosasnas et al., 2017; Jacobson et al., 2017), even this association with slow speed in younger children is small and hardly convincing of it being the core deficit in SCT, as its name clearly implies. Furthermore, others (Bauermeister et al., 2012) did not replicate this finding of slow perceptual–motor or processing speed, despite studying children. Again, replication of such findings is essential before one can have confidence in their linkage to SCT. The meta-analysis of SCT research by Becker, Leopold, and colleagues (2016) likewise concluded that the neurocognitive research on SCT is too scant to draw any firm conclusions.

Only a few studies using psychometric tests of EF specifically have been done with individuals selected for SCT. Unlike ADHD, results intimate that SCT is not as serious and pervasive a disorder of EF, if it involves psychometrically assessed EF at all (Bauermeister et al., 2012; Wahlsted & Bohlin, 2010). In contrast, research is ubiquitous showing that in ADHD, for instance, there are deficits on tests of inhibition and WM, especially nonverbal WM (Frazier et al., 2004; Hervey et al., 2004; Willcutt et al., 2005; Willcutt, 2015). In contrast, this is not seen in SCT; research shows that it is ADHD inattention that is most closely linked to impaired EF test performance. When covaried out of analyses of SCT effects on EF, the result is often one of nonsignificance (Bauermeister et al., 2012; Camprodon-Rosanas et al., 2017a). But the research here is so limited as to preclude any firm conclusions being drawn. Moreover, EF tests have low or no ecological validity and low or no relationships to various domains of impairment, in contrast to ratings of EF (Barkley, 2012b; Barkley & Fischer, 2011; Barkley & Murphy, 2010). And so EF tests cannot serve as the gold or sole standard for examining EF deficits in SCT (or any other disorder). Given their greater ecological validity and predictive power for impairment, EF ratings may provide a different pattern of results for SCT than do EF tests.

Just a few studies have used EF ratings to study individuals with SCT. For instance, my own large studies (Barkley, 2012a, 2013) used my rating scale of EF in daily life with large, epidemiologically derived samples of children and adults having SCT, ADHD, or both. Results for the childhood survey showed that SCT had only very weak relationships to four of the five EF deficit dimensions (<1% shared variance) when statistically controlling for its association with ADHD symptoms, especially the inattention dimension. On one dimension (Planning and Problem-Solving) there was a slightly higher contribution (<5%) after such statistical control. A more recent study of adults with ADHD likewise found that SCT symptoms contributed primarily to the self-organization dimension of EF ratings but not to the other dimensions, once ADHD symptoms were statistically controlled (Leikauf & Solanto, 2017). A study of preschoolers similarly found that parent- and teacher-rated SCT symptoms in the children were not related to ratings of EF in daily life (Tamm, Brenner, et al., 2018). And as explained in Chapter 3 of this manual, when SCT symptoms are factor-analyzed with ratings of EF in daily life, the two dimensions of SCT merge as being distinct from those of EF. This is not the case for ADHD symptoms, which can be found to cross-load onto dimensions of EF rather than forming separate dimensions from them. Again, this implies that ADHD is very much a disorder of EF, whereas SCT is not.

Several studies of college students (Becker et al., 2017; Jarrett, Rapport, Rondon, & Becker, 2014; Wood, Lewandowski, Lovett, & Antshel, 2017) did find some unique contribution of SCT symptoms to some dimensions of EF in daily life independent of ADHD inattention, but typically of a much smaller magnitude than is the case for ADHD inattention. The only exception is in the self-regulation of emotion: Becker et al. (2017) found that SCT symptoms made an equal contribution compared to the two dimensions of ADHD, whereas Jarrett et al. (2014) found that only SCT made such a contribution, controlling for ADHD inattention. This may be the case for adults with SCT symptoms, as was also found in my own U.S. survey of adults, but that was not the case in the survey of U.S. children. So, there may be some age-related changes in this relationship worth further study. Overall, it is the inattentive dimension of ADHD that contributes to the vast majority of variance across most EF dimensions on EF rating scales, with the hyperactive–impulsive dimension accounting for a lesser but still significant degree of variance, especially on the EF dimensions of Self-Restraint (inhibition) and Emotional Self-Regulation. From these results, it seems that SCT is not nearly as much of a disorder of EF, if it is at all, as is ADHD, which is massively so on such ratings. Indeed, ADHD inattention symptoms account for 8–20 times as much variance in most dimensions of EF ratings than do SCT symptoms.

Using a different rating scale of EF, Becker and Langberg (2014) also found a smaller contribution of SCT to the metacognitive factor on the Behavior Rating Inventory of Executive Functioning, in comparison to the inattentive symptoms of ADHD. So did Jimenez and colleagues, even after controlling for ADHD inattention (Jimenez, Ballabriga, Martin, Arrufat, & Giacobo, 2013).

A small link of SCT to EF-like problems was also evident in the study by Langberg and colleagues (Langberg, Becker, & Dvorsky, 2014), but only for parent-reported organizational problems. Yet only ADHD inattention symptoms linked up with organizational problems, as rated by teachers. It is possible that problems with certain aspects of WM may be weakly related or possibly secondary to the cognitive SCT daydreaming dimension. I believe those WM/organizational problems hardly compare to the more severe and pervasive EF deficits so evident in ratings of daily life for children and adults with ADHD (Barkley, 2012a, 2013) and that correlate so much more strongly with ADHD inattention symptoms. Moreover, it is clear across all of these studies utilizing EF rating scales that SCT has no significant association with EF inhibitory problems, whereas those inhibitory problems are substantial in ADHD.

Overlap of ADHD and SCT

In the majority of research on SCT, samples were selected from among children referred to clinics for concerns about ADHD; indeed, in some a diagnosis of some type of ADHD (via DSM-IV criteria) was the starting point. This selection process can automatically make it seem as if SCT were highly associated with, and hence a subtype of, ADHD in the results of such research if any differences emerge at all. It also means one cannot study the overlap or independence of the disorders, given the confounding starting point of case selection. In contrast, if SCT cases are selected specifically from general population or general outpatient clinic samples, there is the opportunity to investigate SCT independently of ADHD, and so the comorbidity between the two could be studied. I did so in my two national surveys (Barkley, 2012a, 2013), wherein I found that more than half (59%) of the children qualifying for a research diagnosis of SCT also met research criteria for having ADHD. Markovich-Pilon et al. (2017) likewise found a high rate of ADHD (40%) in Canadian children referred to an ADHD clinic who were subsequently classified as having high levels of SCT symptoms. But this finding did not differ significantly from the rate (29%) found in those referred children rated low in SCT symptoms, perhaps due to low statistical power in the study design. A few studies suggest that it is among those ADHD subtypes having significant inattention symptoms, rather than with the predominantly hyperactive–impulsive type, that one is most likely to find the overlap with SCT (Garner et al., 2010; Penny et al., 2009; Skirbekk et al., 2011). In my survey, only 39% of the children qualifying for ADHD of any type also qualified for SCT. Again, these findings agree with prior studies of children (Garner et al., 2010; Hartman et al., 2004) and adults (Barkley, 2012a). For instance, one survey of U.S. adults (Barkley, 2012a) found that 5.8% of the sample met criteria for high SCT symptoms. Approximately half (54%) of those participants qualifying for SCT had ADHD, yet nearly half did not. Similarly, approximately half of individuals qualifying for ADHD of any type (46%) also qualified for SCT. It seems to me that the relationship of SCT to ADHD evident in these findings is one of comorbidity between two relatively distinct but related or partially coupled disorders, such as exists between anxiety and depression, and not one of subtyping within a single shared disorder. More research will help clarify if this distinction is, in fact, the case.

Patterns of Comorbidity

SCT symptoms are often linked to elevated ratings of *internalizing symptoms* generally than are ADHD symptoms (Bauermeister et al., 2012; Becker & Langberg, 2013; Becker et al., 2014; Capdevila-Brophy et al., 2012; Carlson & Mann, 2002; Garner et al., 2010; Hartman et al., 2004; Penny et al., 2009; Smith & Langberg, 2017), especially the Slow dimension (Smith & Langberg, 2017). This is so even after controlling for ADHD symptoms (Bauermeister et al., 2012; Becker & Langberg, 2013; Becker, Langberg, Luebbe, Dvorsky, & Flannery, 2014; Burns et al., 2013; Jacobson et al., 2017; Lee et al., 2013; Penny et al., 2009; Willcutt et al., 2013). Among adolescents with ADHD, self-report of SCT was more strongly predictive of internalizing symptoms than were parent reports, which better predicted academic impairment (Smith & Langberg, 2017). This linkage of SCT to internalizing symptoms is undoubtedly one of the most reliable findings in the literature on SCT in child, teen, and adult samples. When the inverse is done, such that SCT symptoms are statistically removed, the inattention dimension of ADHD may be less or even unrelated to internalizing symptoms (Lee et al., 2013; Penny et al., 2009) or even to ratings of social problems (Becker et al., 2014).

The relationships of SCT to *anxiety* and *depression* are positive (Lee et al., 2013), not surprisingly, given that the latter two conditions are often combined in ratings of internalizing symptoms. SCT may predict both of these internalizing dimensions (anxiety, depression) even after controlling for the overlap of the latter dimensions with each other (Becker et al., 2014). The association with depression may be stronger than that with anxiety (Cortes et al., 2017) and remains even after controlling for parental internalizing dimensions, as was done by Becker et al. (2013). Although a few exceptions exist in this literature (Burns et al., 2013; Harrington & Waldman, 2010; Wahlstedt & Bohlin, 2010), the weight of the evidence finds SCT to be more closely related to internalizing symptoms (anxiety, depression, withdrawal) than is ADHD (Becker, Leopold, et al., 2016; Becker et al., 2017). There is a pattern here of a double dissociation between the two disorders in their linkage to internalizing symptoms that is evidence that they are distinct conditions from each other, not subtypes of a common disorder.

There is a lack of association of SCT with *oppositional defiant disorder* (ODD; Barkley, 2013). Furthermore, there is more recent evidence that the relationships may be negative ones when ADHD inattention is removed statistically in the analyses (Cortes et al., 2017). So it can be reasoned that SCT also would have little or no associations with conduct disorder (Cortes et al., 2017), substance use disorders, or adult antisocial personality disorder. That is because all of these risks are linked, to varying degrees, with ODD or the hyperactive–impulsive symptom dimension of ADHD, with which SCT is unassociated. Further evidence for this lack of, or even negative association with, externalizing disorders is evident in a study using direct observations of disciplinary actions (time-outs) received on an inpatient unit (Becker et al., 2014). Such disciplinary actions, often instituted for disruptive or aggressive behavior, were positively linked to the hyperactive–impulsive symptoms of ADHD but negatively associated with SCT symptom severity. This finding is yet another double dissociation supporting the distinctiveness of SCT from ADHD.

One prior study examined the relationship of SCT versus ADHD to specific professional diagnoses of *17 different learning, developmental, and psychiatric disorders,* as reported by parents asked to identify the past professional diagnoses their children had received (Barkley, 2013). This research found that both SCT and ADHD were associated with elevated rates of comorbidity for 11 of the 17 disorders. But SCT was not associated with higher rates of reading or math disorders, hearing impairment, ODD, anxiety, or bipolar disorder diagnoses than the controls. ADHD was linked to higher rates for all of these disorders except hearing impairments. Unlike ADHD, the SCT group had a higher rate of depression than either the controls or those with ADHD, consistent with other studies already cited that found such an association with ratings of depression. The comorbidity of ADHD and SCT was associated with higher rates of comorbidity for most disorders than was either disorder alone. This finding implies an additive effect of SCT and ADHD when they exist together, as if each were a distinct disorder that rendered greater risks when comorbid. Or this pattern could have arisen merely as a function of symptom severity: That is, individuals with comorbid disorders had more symptoms of both disorders than was the case for each specific disorder group.

Even so, another study using Canadian children referred to an ADHD clinic did not find any differences in rates of comorbidity between the children with high versus low SCT symptoms (Markovich-Pilon et al., 2017). This finding is in contrast to the repeated linkage of SCT with internalizing symptoms generally and depression, as noted above. Perhaps it results from a referral bias, however, as clinic-referred children are more likely to have comorbid disorders than are nonreferred children identified as disordered in epidemiological samples (Angold, Costello, & Erkanli, 1999).

One recent study evaluated the extent to which SCT and ADHD symptoms were related to dimensions of *psychopathy* in a large sample ($N = 198$) of inpatient child mental health admissions (Raiker et al., 2015). The two dimensions of psychopathy (psychopathy–impulsivity and narcissism) mediated the linkage between ADHD symptoms and social problems, whereas the symptoms of SCT were unrelated to psychopathy after controlling for their overlap with ADHD.

Domains of Impairment

For a condition to rise to the level of being a mental disorder, there must be evidence of impairment or harm (adverse consequences) to the individual from those symptoms (American Psychiatric Association, 2013). We can think of symptoms as the cognitive, emotional, and behavioral expressions of a disorder, whereas impairment represents the consequences that flow from such symptoms.

Social Functioning

Studies of individuals with SCT symptoms have routinely shown them linked to social problems generally and to social withdrawal specifically (Becker & Langberg, 2013; Becker et al., 2014; Burns et al., 2013; Capdevila-Brophy et al., 2012; Camprodon-Rosanas et al., 2017b; Garner et al., 2010; Marshall et al., 2013; Willcutt et al., 2013), even in the presence of high ADHD inattention symptoms (Capdevila-Brophy et al., 2012) or after controlling for the overlap of ADHD inattention symptoms with those of SCT (Becker, Burns, Schmitt, et al., 2017). Such findings may be even more apparent in teacher than in parent ratings (Bauermeister et al., 2012; Becker & Langberg, 2013). This may be one of the most well-documented associations of SCT with any domain of impairment (Becker, Leopold, et al., 2016), and it differs markedly from the relationship of ADHD to social aggression and peer rejection (McQuade & Hoza, 2015).

Mikami and colleagues (Mikami, Huang-Pollack, Pfiffner, McBurnett, & Hangai, 2007) have provided the only study to date involving detailed observations of the social interactions of children with SCT, using a simulated chat room with children with ADHD and controls. They statistically controlled for ADHD type, IQ, reading ability, and typing skill in their analyses. SCT was noted to independently predict fewer total responses in the chat room, less perception of subtle social cues, less memory for the conversation, and a smaller proportion of hostile responses. While these findings agree with the more general findings that individuals with SCT are more socially withdrawn, they also suggest a role of SCT in attention and an encoding dysfunction that accounts for impairment in critical social behaviors that are of a different sort than seen ADHD (social intrusion, aggression, bossiness, excessive speech, etc.).

Noteworthy is the finding that the association of SCT to social impairment or withdrawal remains even after statistically removing ADHD symptoms as well as those of ODD, conduct disorder, generalized anxiety disorder, major depressive disorder, and IQ (Becker et al., 2016). SCT and the inattention dimension of ADHD both contribute to variance in the presence of social problems and apparently peer neglect, yet their contributions are independent or additive, not redundant (Burns et al., 2013; Willcutt et al., 2013). Similarly, the study by Becker et al. (2013) found that the positive association of SCT with general social problems was apparently not due to disruptive social problems, given the association noted above with significantly lower rates of discipline in inpatient children. This relationship of SCT to social withdrawal persists even after controlling for demographic factors and comorbidity (Becker, Leopold, et al., 2016). Thus SCT contributes unique variance to certain areas of social impairment independent of other disorders, including ADHD.

Academic Functioning

Bauermeister et al. (2012) found that both SCT and ADHD inattention were each significantly and independently associated with lower academic achievement scores on testing after controlling for the other set of symptoms, whereas hyperactive–impulsive symptoms showed no such relationship. Markovich-Pilon et al. (2017) also found a weak negative relationship of SCT symptoms with academic achievement tests ($r = -.22$), albeit barely significant, but only for teacher-rated SCT symptoms. In contrast, three studies (Becker & Langberg, 2013; Langberg et al., 2014; Watabe, Owens, Evans, & Brandt, 2013) either did not find an association of SCT symptoms with academic achievement test performances after controlling for IQ and ADHD symptoms, or found it to be rather weak. Again, the source of the ratings of SCT may account for this disparity in results across studies on achievement tests.

A few studies found that SCT symptoms may be uniquely associated with deficient math performance (Bauermeister et al., 2012; Tamm, Garner, et al., 2016). Again, the source of the ratings may be relevant to such findings, in that they may be more evident in teacher- than in parent-rated SCT symptoms.

Others have found some measures of SCT symptoms to be uniquely linked to problems with writing (but not reading). However, once again these relationships varied depending on source (parent vs. teacher ratings; Tamm, Garner, et al., 2016) with stronger associations evident in teacher- than in parent-rated SCT symptoms, just as Markovich-Pilon et al. (2017) found (above).

In contrast to these mixed results using academic test performances, far stronger associations have been found for SCT symptoms when ratings of academic impairment are used (Burns et al., 2013; Tamm, Garner, et al., 2016). Like Burns et al. (2013), Camprodon-Rosanas et al. (2017b) noted this same relationship in Spanish children. Likewise, Flannery, Luebbe, and Becker (2017) found SCT symptoms to be uniquely linked to poorer study skills and globally rated educational impairment. Such relationships are evident even after controlling for ADHD inattention symptoms in the preceding and other studies (Becker, Burns, Schmitt, et al., 2017). The results of the study by Tamm, Garner, et al. (2016) indicate that it is the Slow or Sluggish dimension of SCT symptoms and not the Daydreamy/Spacey dimension that is related to academic impairment ratings. Smith and Langberg (2017) found the same result in a study of teens with ADHD, particularly for parent ratings of that SCT Slow dimension. In contrast, youth self-report in that study was more strongly predictive of internalizing symptoms. Further evidence of academic functioning difficulties being linked to high SCT symptoms comes from a recent study by Shelton and colleagues (Shelton, Addison, & Hartung, 2017). They found SCT symptoms to be uniquely associated with certain self-regulated learning (SRL) strategies in college students apart from the SRL deficits linked to ADHD symptoms. Likewise, Becker and colleagues found a relationship of SCT symptoms to poor academic functioning in college students (Becker et al., 2014).

The reason for the differences in results concerning academic functioning is obvious. It is the type of measurement of academic functioning and achievement being used in the study. Ratings of academic functioning in daily life are linked in specific and unique ways to SCT symptoms, independent of those related to ADHD, which may not be evident when psychometric tests of certain academic achievement skills are studied for their relationship to SCT.

Why else might there be a disparity across these studies besides measurement type? It may arise from the fact that some studies selected their samples for ADHD first and then within such samples, examined those high and low in SCT symptoms or examined the relationship of SCT to other correlates. This method can contaminate any findings for SCT with those results related to ADHD. Even so, when symptoms of ADHD are statistically removed, SCT appears to add unique variance to the prediction of academic problems (Barkley, 2013; Becker, Leopold, et al., 2016; Becker, Burns, Schmitt, et al., 2017; Smith & Langberg, 2017) and may make unique contributions to written language, organization problems, and homework specifically beyond the contribution of ADHD inattention symptoms (Langberg, Becker, & Dvorsky, 2014; Marshall et al., 2013; Willcutt et al., 2013).

Sleep

Given that problems with alertness, remaining awake, and even daytime sleepiness have been used as symptoms to index the presence of SCT (Penny et al., 2009), it is not surprising that the condition has been challenged for being a mere proxy of hypersomnia, or excess sleepiness. So, for SCT to be established as a unique condition from other psychiatric or psychological problems, its relative independence from daytime drowsiness and nighttime sleep problems needs to be established. Several recent studies have now done so. A study of 7,346 clinic-referred children evaluated this relationship (Koriakin et al., 2015). Parent and teacher ratings were used to assess ADHD, SCT, anxiety, and depression symptoms along with parent reports of sleep problems. Controlling for ADHD, anxiety, depression, age, and medication status, the study showed only difficulty waking was significantly related to SCT, but only parent-rated and not teacher-rated. This relationship was primarily with the Sleepy/Sluggish dimension of SCT, as one might expect. Another recent study examined 325 children referred to a sleep disorders clinic at a major children's hospital (Becker, Garner, et al., 2016). It found that SCT was weakly linked to most measures of sleep but moderately correlated (.33–.53) with daytime sleepiness, after controlling for child demographic factors, corroborating the Koriakin et al. (2015) findings. Further corroboration comes from a recent study of children referred to a Canadian ADHD clinic (Markovich-Pilon et al., 2017), in which, again, only parent-rated SCT, but not teacher-rated, was associated with daytime sleepiness, but not with nighttime sleeping problems or duration. Thus, only parent-rated SCT symptoms in children, especially along the Sleepy/Sluggish dimension, may share about 10–30% of variance with daytime sleepiness. This is not true of teacher-rated SCT. The finding for parent ratings is not surprising, given the inclusion of some items pertaining to sleepy/drowsy in SCT ratings.

A study of college students (Becker, Luebbe, & Langberg, 2014) likewise found a significant association of SCT symptoms, but not ADHD inattention, with poorer sleep quality and increased nighttime sleep disturbance. Yet both SCT and ADHD inattention were associated with greater daytime dysfunction, above and beyond those nighttime sleep disturbances. In contrast, ADHD hyperactivity symptoms were linked to poorer sleep quality, longer sleep latency, shorter sleep duration, and more use of sleep medications. But the small degree of the association in these studies, even if significant, means that SCT is not simply serving as a proxy for hypersomnia, daytime sleepiness, or sleeping difficulties, although it may be comorbid with, and possibly contributory to, both nighttime sleep problems and daytime dysfunction.

Driving

Only one study to date has examined the relationship of SCT to driving problems (Garner et al., 2016) experienced by 16- to 18-year-old adolescents with a history of chronically short sleep (5–7 hours). Results found that parent-reported (but not self-reported) symptoms of SCT were significantly associated with driving violations (self-reported). In contrast, ADHD symptoms show a more marked and pervasive adverse relationship to various measures of driving performance and outcomes (Barkley, 2015c). Of interest to clinicians is that a treatment program intended to increase sleep time in these adolescents resulted in both a reduction in SCT symptoms and in fewer driving problems.

Global Impairment

In addition to social and academic domains, my own national surveys of children and adults included a measure of 15 domains of impairment (Barkley, 2012a, 2013). Individuals were sorted into those who had SCT only, those with ADHD only, those with both conditions, and the remainder serving as the community control group. Individuals with SCT were more impaired in all domains than control cases, having their greatest difficulties in community–leisure domains more than in home–school (work) domains. In contrast, although individuals with ADHD were also impaired across all domains, their greatest difficulties occurred in home–school domains. Moreover, ADHD was associated with more pervasive impairment. That is, both ADHD groups (alone and combined with SCT) experienced impairment in at least twice as many of the 15 domains as did those with SCT. The results also showed that ADHD symptom dimensions, especially inattention, contributed markedly more variance to impairment in the home–school domains than did hyperactive–impulsive or SCT dimensions. By contrast, the hyperactive–impulsive dimension contributed more variance to community–leisure impairments, as did SCT, but to a far lesser extent. When considering individual domains among the 15 rated, SCT was not found to be more impairing than ADHD in educational settings, at least as rated by parents, consistent with other research discussed previously. When ADHD and SCT symptoms were regressed onto the community–leisure and home–school impairment summary scores, results found that both contributed uniquely to impairment, although ADHD accounted for a greater proportion of variance in each summary score. Hence, in children, SCT is a less impairing disorder than ADHD, though hardly benign.

The adult survey (Barkley, 2012a) also used a rating scale of impairment in 15 domains more appropriate to adults. Both the SCT-only and ADHD-only groups were more impaired than the control group but did not differ in this respect in overall mean impairment. A somewhat different pattern was evident for the percentage of domains in which impairment occurred (pervasiveness). Here, both of the ADHD groups (ADHD alone, ADHD+SCT) were impaired in more domains than was the SCT-only group and the control group. The results further revealed that the SCT-only group was impaired in more domains than the control group of adults, but not to the degree evident in the ADHD groups. These results are consistent with the more recent large-scale study of college students by Becker and colleagues (2017), in that impairment is certainly linked to SCT in distinct ways, than is ADHD but may not be so impairing as ADHD. A separate study of college students also found SCT to be uniquely linked to global impairment as well as to the specific domains of education, work, money and finances, managing household tasks and chores, community activities, and social situations, despite controlling for ADHD symptoms and anxiety and depression ratings (Flannery et al., 2017).

It is noteworthy that in both of my large U.S. studies, when comorbid, ADHD+SCT disorders were additive in their impact on impairment ratings. That is, the combination of disorders resulted in far more severe impairment and more domains of impairment than either disorder alone.

Quality of Life

Combs and colleagues have also studied the linkage of SCT to some aspects of impairment in large adult community samples (Combs, Canu, Broman, & Nieman, 2013; Combs, Canu, Broman-Fulks, Rocheleau, & Nieman, 2012). In one study (Combs et al., 2013), the authors evaluated the contribution of both ADHD and SCT symptoms to quality of life (QOL). Findings indicated that each set of symptoms contributed unique variance to negative QOL ratings, after controlling for the other set of symptoms as well as for anxiety, depression, and some demographic factors. The second study (Combs et al., 2012) found much the same results for the association of ADHD and SCT with self-reported stress in adults. All of the preceding research suggests that SCT is associated with distinct impairments in various domains of functioning from those associated with ADHD and contributes unique effects to impairment beyond that accounted for by ADHD.

Etiology

Very few studies have been done on the etiologies of SCT. A study by Moruzzi, Rijsdijk, and Battaglia (2014) examined the heritability of SCT using a very small set of items. SCT was substantially though moderately heritable, with genetic factors accounting for the majority of variance in symptoms. However, a greater proportion of its variance was attributable to nonshared environmental factors than was the case for ADHD symptoms, which were even more substantially accounted for by genetic factors. And SCT shared about half of its genetic contribution with that of ADHD, implying some shared underlying genetic contributions but some unique to each disorder as well. Given the limited SCT item set, findings might have been different (larger heritability factor) had a longer and hence more reliable SCT scale been employed (because unreliability of measurement is clustered with the nonshared environment estimate).

Several studies observed a link between SCT symptoms and exposure to environmental toxins. One study observed that SCT was associated with prenatal alcohol exposure (Graham et al., 2013). Another noted the association of this symptom dimension with maternal smoking during pregnancy and also secondhand smoke exposure after birth (Camprodon-Rosanas, Ribas-Fitó, et al., 2017). It has also been seen as a treatment-emergent side effect, along with lower IQ and lower academic achievement, in individuals with acute lymphoblastic leukemia (Reeves et al., 2007).

One neuroimaging study has been reported in which SCT symptoms were more strongly associated with abnormal activity in posterior networks related to impaired orienting and shifting of attention, as opposed to abnormalities in frontal–parietal (executive) networks so often evident in ADHD (Fassbender, Krafft, & Schweitzer, 2015). The findings support a degree of differentiation between SCT symptoms and ADHD symptoms in the performance of controlled cognitive activities. Yet one study doesn't make a definitive conclusion here.

And so it seems that, like ADHD, SCT may turn out to have multiple etiologies. Most causes may fall in the realm of neurobiological and genetic factors, perhaps less strongly than does ADHD. We sorely need more research that uses neuroimaging as well as more behavioral genetic and molecular genetic studies on the nature of SCT in comparison to other disorders, especially ADHD. However, researchers must take care to control for the overlap of SCT with ADHD. Not doing so will contaminate any findings with ADHD-related results.

What Is the Underlying Mental Dysfunction in SCT?

We simply do not know. It is possible that SCT represents a dysfunction in the focus/execute component of attention in Mirsky's (1996) model of attention components. It is also possible that SCT is a form of hypersomnia or arousal disorder, given that some dimensions of SCT identified in past research include symptoms of sleepiness, low arousal or energy, or drowsiness (Penny et al., 2009). But this seems unlikely in view of recent evidence in college students that although both SCT and ADHD were significantly associated with daytime sleepiness, sleepiness formed a distinct factor from those representing SCT and ADHD (Langberg, Becker, Dvorsky, & Luebbe, 2014). So SCT is not just another label or proxy for hypersomnia, but it does have a significant association with daytime sleepiness, even after controlling for ADHD, anxiety, and depression symptoms (Langberg, Becker, Dvorsky, & Luebbe, 2014).

Could SCT be a form of pathological mind wandering or maladaptive daydreaming (Adams et al., 2010)? The fact that the only neuroimaging study that linked SCT symptoms to the posterior regions that are implicated in the default mode network, and that this network has a close association with mind wandering (Christoff, Irving, Fox, Spreng, & Andrews-Hanna, 2016), suggests this possibility. Research shows that mind wandering is commonplace and advantageous under certain conditions. It arises when a primary task being performed demands little EF capacity and thus allows the contemplative or problem-solving capacity of the EF system to focus on more salient personal concerns. The latter then becomes a secondary task that is engaged while the individual performs the relatively automatic actions toward familiar goals (primary task) in the environment (Smallwood & Schooler, 2006). When poorly regulated, however, mind wandering can lead to adverse effects when performing EF tasks (perhaps due to reduced meta-awareness or self-monitoring of goal pursuit, diminished WM capacity available for pursing the external goals, etc.) (Smallwood & Schooler, 2006). Excessive mind wandering also can adversely affect academic performance (Smallwood, Fishman, & Schooler, 2007). It would seem to be worthwhile for future research to investigate this possible association of SCT with pathological mind wandering.

There are still other possibilities concerning the underlying nature of SCT. For instance, SCT could arise from a ruminative/obsessional disorder, perhaps being a milder variant of obsessive–compulsive disorder (OCD). Excessive and recurrent focusing on maladaptive thoughts might well lead to an attention problem resembling SCT. The same could be said for the attention problems evident in posttraumatic stress disorder (PTSD). Or SCT could represent a deficit in motivation in which the person lacks not only energy but also initiative or self-motivation. I think that is unlikely, given that research has not linked SCT to deficits in self-motivation, as reflected on EF rating scales by children or adults, once the overlap with ADHD symptoms is statistically removed (Barkley, 2012a, 2013; Becker et al., 2017).

Diagnosing SCT

During the initial evaluation of a child or adult, the suspicion of SCT can arise when there are complaints of inattention in the context of low or no symptoms of hyperactivity or impulsivity and when symptoms of passivity, hypoactivity, and even social withdrawal are evident (Saxbe & Barkley, 2014). Clinicians can then use rating scales that directly assess SCT symptoms (see Barkley, 2011a, for adults and the BSCTS-CA for children) to evaluate the extent to which such symptoms are statistically abnormal relative to population norms, thus revealing the extent of developmental deviance.

There is no official set of diagnostic criteria for SCT. My own research (Barkley, 2013) suggests that if parents endorse at least three or more of the 12 symptoms of SCT on the BSCTS-CA rating scale discussed earlier, and they occur at least "often," this profile would represent the 93rd percentile in the population. That percentile, which is a traditional index of clinical significance and statistical deviance, combined with evidence of impairment from the symptoms, could be used (for the time being) as unofficial diagnostic criteria for SCT in children. It would identify about 5% of the U.S. child population as having this condition.

In the case of an adult, the symptom threshold would be five out of the nine symptoms used in my study of adults (Barkley, 2012a) and reflected on an adult SCT rating scale (Barkley, 2011a). When coupled with evidence of impairment in one or more major life activities, such as may be shown on normed rating scales of impairment (Barkley, 2011b, 2012c), one can make an unofficial diagnosis of SCT.

Treatment of SCT

As with the etiology of SCT, only a few studies have investigated possible treatments for SCT, all in children. Early studies on stimulants (methylphenidate [MPH]) for treating individuals with ADHD inattentive type did not find them to be particularly effective in improving the inattention linked to SCT (Milich et al., 2001), although they were not harmful either. My own study found a modest positive response to MPH, mainly at low doses, but with only 20% of individuals remaining on this medication after a double-blind, placebo-controlled trial. That low percentage contrasted sharply with the fact that the vast majority of children with ADHD combined type stayed on that medication and their degree of improvement was greater than that of children with ADHD inattentive type, who also showed SCT symptoms (Barkley, DuPaul, & McMurray, 1991). But no stimulant medication studies have been done specifically with individuals with SCT. Even so, recent research (Froehlich et al., in press) reported that higher SCT symptoms predicted a poorer response to MPH, consistent with the earlier studies on ADD–H or the predominantly inattentive type of ADHD.

Only one study to date has examined a nonstimulant ADHD medication for treating SCT symptoms specifically (Wietecha et al., 2013). The researchers found that the norepinephrine reuptake inhibitor *atomoxetine* was effective at reducing SCT symptoms in patients having both ADHD and dyslexia, ADHD only, and dyslexia only. The reduction in SCT symptoms remained evident even after statistically controlling for the overlap of ADHD symptoms and also improved SCT symptoms in the group with dyslexia only (McBurnett et al., 2017).

What other medications might work to treat SCT? Given its overlap with anxiety and depression, perhaps selective serotonin reuptake inhibitors (SSRIs) could be a possible treatment. Would an activating antidepressant (e.g., fluoxetine, sertraline, venlafaxine, or bupropion) reduce the observed sluggishness and boost alertness? Some clinicians have used Luvox (fluvoxamine, which functions as an SSRI) for management of pathological mind wandering, given its effects on obsessional thinking, but it is not clear that such thinking is the case in SCT. Given that SCT is associated with hypersomnia or daytime sleepiness, should one consider investigating the use of anti-narcoleptics, such as Modafinil? It seems to me that the alpha-2 agonist guanfacine XR, used for management of ADHD, might be worth investigating for SCT, but its side effects of sleepiness could be counterproductive in view of the sluggish/sleepy features seen in SCT. There is great opportunity for research here to explore possible medications for the management of this condition.

Just two studies of behavior modification methods have been conducted to date, and these were done with individuals with predominantly inattentive ADHD, many of whom had SCT. The results indicated a good response of children with SCT symptoms to traditional home and school behavior management methods when targeted to the specific symptoms of SCT (Pfiffner et al., 2007). Although it did not use SCT cases specifically, one study of social skills training found that children with ADHD inattention type (who are more likely to have SCT) improved more in their assertion skills than did those with ADHD combined type (Antshel & Remer, 2003). Yet no children with either type of ADHD improved in other domains of social skills. Cognitive-behavioral therapy (CBT) has not been shown to be useful for ADHD (Abikoff, 1985), but it has proven useful for cases of anxiety and/or depression (Cuijpers, Berking, Andersson, Quigley, Kleiboer, & Dobson, 2013). I believe it may be worth exploring as a possible intervention for SCT, given the higher-than-expected comorbidity between these disorders. In view of the distinct symptoms and impairments of SCT relative to ADHD, treatments for ADHD cannot be automatically assumed to work for SCT nor can those treatments that have failed for ADHD be thus ruled out for SCT.

Conclusions

- SCT is an impairment of attention in daydreamy, hypoactive-appearing individuals, which first presents in childhood. It is characterized by a cognitive dimension of symptoms, comprising daydreaming, sleepiness, staring, "spaciness," and mental fogginess and confusion, along with a motor dimension of slow movement, hypoactivity, lethargy, and passivity.
- The symptom dimensions forming SCT are distinct from, yet partially correlated with, those forming ADHD, especially its inattention dimension.
- To avoid giving offense to patients having the condition and their families, as well as to avoid implying that the cognitive deficit in SCT is known, the condition should be called by a more benign label, such as CDD.
- The history of SCT in the medical literature probably dates back to Alexander Crichton in 1798 or, at the very least, to 1984, as found in research exploring the validity of ADD–H created in DSM-III.
- At this time SCT exists only as a research entity that has yet to debut in diagnostic literature.
- SCT is associated with significant impairment, most reliably in social impairment, primarily social withdrawal. It also makes some contribution to difficulties with academic performance in children, and by adulthood even more so. In adults it is associated with impairment in occupational functioning.
- SCT is significantly associated with risk for internalizing symptoms, especially depression, and likely anxiety as well.
- It has no, or even a negative, relationship to ODD (and hence likely has no, or even a negative, relationship to conduct disorder, substance use disorders, or antisocial personality disorder).
- The etiologies of SCT are not well studied, but some evidence suggests a strong heritability to the disorder, though not as much as is seen in ADHD. SCT may also be associated with fetal alcohol exposure and with the treatment of acute lymphoblastic leukemia. Perhaps abnormal activity in the brain's default mode network may be linked to SCT, as one study suggests.
- Evidence supports the view that SCT is distinct from ADHD and not a subtype of it, but the two conditions can overlap in nearly half of all cases of each.
- Future diagnostic taxonomies, such as the DSM, should create a higher-order category of attention disorders under which one would then break out ADHD and SCT as separate, semidistinct conditions, much like what is done now for the supracategory of learning disabilities (LDs), rather than continue the mistaken view that SCT is a subtype of ADHD.
- Very little research has been done on treatments for SCT, so no conclusions concerning its management can be made at this time.

CHAPTER 2

Scale Development, Survey Methods, and Normative Sample

In this chapter the history and initial development of the BSCTS-CA is overviewed, followed by a description of the methods used to collect information on the scale from the normative sample of U.S. parents having children ages 6–17 years.

Developmental History of the BSCTS-CA

The BSCTS-CA was initially developed as part of a national survey assessing ADHD symptoms, EF deficits, and functional impairments in major life activities (see Chapter 1; Barkley, 2012c, 2012d). Items on the BSCTS-CA were constructed from a review of the available literature on items having potential utility in identifying cases of SCT and, in particular, the results of the research of McBurnett et al. (2001) and Penny et al. (2009). As noted in Chapter 1, 14 items were originally identified and included in the national survey of U.S. children, described later. These were (1) daydreaming, (2) trouble staying awake/alert, (3) mentally foggy/easily confused, (4) stares a lot, (5) spacey/mind is elsewhere, (6) lethargic, (7) underactive, (8) slow-moving/sluggish, (9) doesn't process questions or explanations accurately, (10) drowsy/sleepy appearance, (11) apathetic/withdrawn, (12) lost in thoughts, (13) slow to complete tasks, and (14) lacks initiative/effort fades. The last two of those items loaded as highly on the ADHD inattention symptom dimension as they did on the SCT dimension in subsequent factor analysis of the items, and so they would not be of much value in differentiating SCT from ADHD. Therefore, those two items were eliminated from further inclusion in the final version of the BSCTS-CA, provided in the Appendix to this manual.

As reported in Chapter 1, 10 of the 13 items identified in the meta-analysis by Becker, Leopold, et al. (2016) and shown in Table 1.1 are contained on the BSCTS-CA form. Furthermore, 8 of the 10 items from the adult validation study (Becker et al., 2017) likewise appear on this form. So the BSCTS-CA clearly captures the majority of the most valid and useful SCT symptoms identified as optimal for differentiating SCT from ADHD, as well as other disorders. That is true even though the scale was developed prior to these two research reports.

The BSCTS-CA scale items are derived from parents' ratings of the degree of symptom frequency they believe their child is experiencing for each symptom, rather than ratings of the appropriate, typical, positive, or normative form of that behavior. The scale was intended for clinical purposes to be used to evaluate the range of symptoms in clinic-referred or high-risk children or adolescents. In that situation, the examiner is faced with the question of the extent to which the complaints about a clinical patient concerning his/her problems are indicative of a mental disorder. The question here is how *typical* or *atypical* are parents' complaints of their child's attention problems, rather than the issue of where does the child place within the distribution of normal variation in symptom functioning in the general population. In other words, the BSCTS-CA approaches the issue of impairment from the standpoint of deficit measurement.

The use of deficit measurement is typical in the development of clinical assessment devices like those used to assess child behavioral problems, such as the Child Behavior Checklist (CBCL) and Behavior Assessment System for Children (BASC). The distribution of such scores is quite different than the more typical bell-shaped curve of the distribution of normal variation in a typical psychological ability, such as intelligence or academic achievement. The score distribution of the deficit measurement tool can be expected to have a highly skewed distribution toward the zero point or low score end on the scale, with a steep fall-off in the percentage of the general population that manifests an increasing degree and frequency of symptoms. Deficit assessment evaluates the likelihood that the complaints of a parent are sufficiently severe or numerous as to place the child or teen significantly outside the distribution of typical complaints for the general population. This is the purpose of the BSCTS-CA: It is a deficit measurement method, not a test of normal variation in a human ability. Hence, its instructions direct the respondent to report the degree of difficulties his/her child experiences, rather than trying to assess the range of normal abilities.

Normative information is *not* available for the interview form of the BSCTS-CA provided in the Appendix. Instead, the form is used for several purposes. One is to obtain more detailed qualitative information on the nature of the SCT symptoms, rated as being clinically significant or impaired, so as to further validate the parent's rating. A second purpose is to accommodate parents who may have problems with literacy and be unable to read and hence unable to complete the written rating scale version.

Methods for Collecting the Normative Sample

The initial 14-item version of the BSCTS-CA was given to a nationally representative sample of 1,922 parents in the United States who had children between the ages of 6 and 17. Instructions were given to the survey company contracted to obtain this national sample to ensure that equal representation of males and females occurred in each of 12 age groups for each of nine regions representing the United States. The company chosen for this task was Knowledge Networks of Menlo Park, California (see *www.knowledgenetworks.org* for more information on the company). Knowledge Networks did so using the web-enabled Knowledge Panel®, a probability-based panel designed to be representative of the U.S. population. Initially, participants were chosen scientifically by a random selection of telephone numbers and residential addresses. Persons in selected households are then invited by telephone or by mail to participate in the web-enabled Knowledge Panel. For those who agree to participate, but do not already have access, Knowledge Networks provides a laptop and ISP connection at no cost. This is a very important factor, because surveying only people who already have computers and Internet connections immediately biases the sample away from one that is representative of the U.S. population. People who already have computers and Internet service are permitted to participate using their own equipment. Panelists then receive unique log-in information for accessing surveys online, and then are sent emails throughout each month inviting them to participate in research. Panelists are paid for their completion of the survey. And those who complete the survey a second time as part of an effort to obtain test–retest reliability on the survey are also paid again. More technical information is available at *www.knowledgenetworks.com/ganp/reviewer-info.html.*

The BSCTS-CA was provided to Knowledge Networks as a rating scale in which respondents were to answer each item using a 4-point Likert scale (1–4), with anchor points being 1 = rarely or not at all, 2 = sometimes, 3 = often, and 4 = very often. The scale was uploaded to an Internet site, and members of the Knowledge Panel were invited to complete them. The interview version was not used in this study. The survey was conducted in August 2011 and was completed within 3 weeks of the initial invitation. The company was contracted to obtain parent-completed scales on at least 1,800 children, broken down into 12 age groups (6, 7, 8, 9, 10, 11, 12, 13, 14, 15, 16, 17) having at least 75 males and 75 females in each age group. A final sample of 1,922 children was obtained.

Knowledge Networks requires that participants be given the option of choosing not to answer a question. In these rare cases, the missing answer was replaced with the response of 1 or "rarely or not at all" so that the remaining data for this participant could be used in the project.

Important to note here is that this sample was not subsequently filtered to remove individuals with a prior history of special education; of taking psychiatric medication; having any psychiatric diagnosis; or who may have had any learning, developmental, neurological, or medical disorders, as occurred in the collection of normative information for other scales. Doing so creates a supernormal comparison group, not a general population sample, and can result in the determination of clinically significant symptoms being found to occur at far lower levels of deviance on the ratings than would be the case had a general population sample, free of such filtering, been used. The BSCTS-CA is based on just such an unfiltered general population sample, so that individual impairment scores on it can be compared to the average, typical, or general person standard. In short, as clinicians we want to know where a given child places in his/her position within the general population of children, not relative to some well-functioning, unimpaired, asymptomatic, non-disordered, and untreated subset of that population.

Demographic Characteristics of the National Sample

The company was originally contracted to obtain completed scales on at least 1,800 children, broken down into 12 age groups (6–17 years), with at least 75 boys and 75 girls in each age group. The company was able to obtain ratings from 1,922 parents with at least 80 boys and 80 girls at each of these years. Initial analyses of the demographic profile showed that the sample was slightly overrepresented with male respondents (fathers) (53% vs. 47% females). It was also somewhat overrepresented with White individuals (74%) compared to the 2000 U.S. Census (69.1%). In addition, it was overrepresented with college-educated (bachelor's degree or higher = 42%) people compared to the U.S. Census (25%). Consequently, the original sample was reduced by 6% (*N* =122) by removing White males having at least a bachelor's degree or higher. Those chosen for removal were proportionately weighted across bachelor's (*N* = 62), master's (*N* = 40), and doctoral degrees (*N* = 20) and equally distributed between male (*N* = 61) and female (*N* = 61) children so as to retain an equal representation of boys and girls at each of the original age levels. The selection of an individual for removal from among those meeting these characteristics was done at random. The final sample used to create the norms reported here therefore consists of 1,800 parents (and their children). This slightly reduced sample is referred to henceforth as the *normative sample.* All further analyses reported in the remainder of this chapter are based on this normative sample.

Age, Sex, and Biological Relationship

The ages of the parents in the normative sample completing the rating scale ranged from 18 to 68 years, with an average of 42.3 years (*SD* = 7.9). The parent respondent reported that 95.3% of the children in this survey had another parent known to them (*N* = 1,715). That parent ranged in age from 21 to 76 years, with a mean age of 42.5 (SD = 7.5). The mean age of the children in the sample was 11.8 years (*SD* = 3.7). The sex of the parent respondent was equally represented, with 50% being fathers (*N* = 900) and 50% being mothers (*N* = 900). Biological parents represented 91% of the sample. The specific breakdown of the status of the parents' biological relationship to the children was biological mother = 46.4%, stepmother = 1.5%, adoptive mother = 1.3%, and foster mother = 0.1%; biological father = 44.8%, stepfather = 3.1%, adoptive father = 1.7%, and foster father = 1.1%.

Education

The breakdown in educational categories for the parent respondents in comparison to the 2000 U.S. Census (*www.census.gov*) is shown below:

Education category	Normative sample %	U.S. Census %
Less than high school	4.1	19.1
High school (diploma or equivalency)	28.1	28.6
Some college, no degree	20.6	21.0
Associate's degree	9.2	6.3
Bachelor's degree	22.6	15.5
Graduate degree	15.4	8.9

The present sample is generally comparable to the U.S. population for the percentage having high school or some college or associate's degree, but has a slight overrepresentation of individuals with a bachelor's degree or graduate degree. Thus the sample contains a lower percentage of those having less than a high school education than is the case for the U.S. Census. As for the educational level of the other parent (nonrespondent), the breakdown was less than high school = 6.6%, high school = 20.6%, some college but no degree = 20.6%, associate's degree = 10.2%, bachelor's degree = 22.8%, or graduate degree = 14.8%. These percentages are very similar to those for the respondent parent. The mean educational level for the children in the sample was 7.4 years (*SD* = 3.5, range = kindergarten [1] to 12th grade [13]) or roughly a mid-sixth-grade education.

Geographic Regions

The geographic distribution of the participants was as follows in comparison to the 2000 U.S. Census:

U.S. geographic region	Normative sample %	U.S. Census %
Northeast	18	19
Midwest	28	23
South	31	36
West	23	22

Thus, the regional representation of the normative sample comes from all regions of the U.S. and appears to approximate that of the adult U.S. population.

Ethnicity

The racial/ethnic breakdown of the normative sample is as follows relative to the 2000 U.S. Census:

Ethnic group	Normative sample %	U.S. Census %
White	73.0	75.1
Black	7.7	12.3
Other (Asian, Native U.S.)	4.3	6.6
Hispanic	12.4	12.5
Multiracial	2.7	2.4

The sample contains members of all major ethnic groups in the United States and appears to approximate that of the U.S. population, except for a somewhat lower representation of Blacks in the normative sample relative to the U.S. Census.

Household Income

The breakdown of the normative sample by income categories follows, again relative to the 2000 U.S. Census:

Income category	Normative sample %	U.S. Census %
Less than $10,000	5.4	9.5
$10,000 to $14,499	2.9	6.3
$15,000 to $24,999	5.5	12.8
$25,000 to $34,999	7.7	12.8
$35,000 to $49,999	11.4	16.5
$50,000 to $74,999	20.4	19.5
$75,000 to $99,999	18.8	10.2
$100,000 to $149,999	18.7	7.7
$150,000+	9.3	4.6

The mean income category was 12.5, which translated to an approximate mean income ranging from $50,000 to $59,999, and the median category was $60,000 to $74,999. This was also the modal income category. The median household income of the United States is $41,994 as of the 2000 U.S. Census. The results suggest this sample of parents has a somewhat higher average household income than that of the U.S. population. However, once again, these figures are not directly comparable, given that the U.S. Census does not provide a breakdown of household income solely for parents within the age range of children used here. It is possible that parents have a somewhat higher mean household income than do individuals who are not parents in the population.

Marital Status of Parents

The marital status of the parents in the normative sample, relative to the parents of children reported in the 2000 U.S. Census, was:

Marital status	Normative sample %	U.S. Census %
Married	81.3	69.0
Separated, divorced, widowed	8.3	19.0
Never married	4.3	11.9

As this table shows, the normative sample has a slightly higher representation of married parents than is the case for parents of children in the U.S. population.

Employment Status of Parents

The employment status of the normative sample was 64.8% working as paid employee, 8.7% self-employed, 1.2% not working/on temporary layoff, 6.8% not working/looking for work, 1.1% retired, 4.5% disabled/not working, and 12.9% not working for other reasons (e.g., housewife or househusband). Approximately 74% of the sample was working. Comparable figures could not be located from the U.S. Census for the age range of parents and children in the normative sample. However, overall employment in the 2000 U.S. Census was 64% for individuals 18 years and older. The employment figure for the normative sample is nearly identical to this figure from the 2000 U.S. Census.

To summarize the demographic characteristics, it appears that the normative sample recruited here reasonably approximates that of the adult U.S. population, as based on the U.S. Census from the year 2000, concerning regional distribution, sex, race/ethnic group, and employment status. It is unclear how this sample compares to the U.S. population in household income because such figures are not readily available from the U.S. Census for parents within this age range having children within the age range of the normative sample. The normative sample has a somewhat higher representation of parents who are married and who are college graduates.

Developmental and Psychiatric Diagnoses of Children

Parents were queried as to whether or not their child had ever received any of the following diagnoses from a professional. Alongside each diagnosis is the percentage of the normative sample that had received such a diagnosis:

Diagnosis	Sample %
Physically disabled (unable to talk or use arms unassisted)	0.3
Language delay	5.0
Delayed motor skills or coordination	3.3

(continued)

Diagnosis	Sample %
Reading disorder or disability	4.2
Math disorder or disability	2.4
Spelling disorder or disability	2.4
Writing disorder or disability	2.3
Other academic learning disorder	1.7
General developmental delay or mental retardation	1.2
Tic disorder or Tourette syndrome	0.6
Deaf or hard of hearing	0.4
Blind or visually impaired	0.6
Seizure disorder or epilepsy	0.8
ADD or ADHD	9.2
ODD	1.6
Conduct disorder	0.3
Any anxiety disorder	3.0
Any depression disorder	1.8
Bipolar disorder or manic–depression	0.8
Autism or autistic spectrum disorder or Asperger syndrome	1.8
Childhood schizophrenia or psychosis	0.1
No diagnosis of any of the above	77.1

The rates for the listed disorders are well within the range found in various epidemiological studies of the U.S. population of children (American Psychiatric Association, 2000, 2013; Mash & Barkley, 2003), except that there appears to be an underrepresentation of children diagnosed with ODD or with conduct disorder. Approximately 23% of the sample had one or more disorders. The results are reasonably consistent with research showing that, on average, 12–13.5% of children ages 6–12 years and 16.5% of children ages 13–18 years have at least one psychiatric disorder (Costello, Egger, & Angold, 2005; Roberts, Attkisson, & Rosenblatt, 1998), typically ranging between 14 and 20% depending on methods used for diagnosis (Brandenburg, Friedman, & Silver, 1990). Some recent studies found an overall prevalence for psychiatric disorders for a 3-month period of 13.5% and a lifetime prevalence throughout a 3-year follow-up during childhood of 36.7% (Costello, Mustillo, Erkanli, Keeler, & Angold, 2003). Add to the average prevalence of 13–16% the percentage of those having intellectual, learning, language, and motor disorders that account for another 10–12% of the population, exclusive of psychiatric disorders (Boyle, Decoufle, & Yeargin-Allsop, 1994; Mash & Barkley, 2003), and one finds that on average 23–29% of the U.S. population of children have at least one developmental, learning, or psychiatric disorder. The overall prevalence of 23% in the present normative sample is therefore a close approximation of the prevalence of these disorders in the U.S. population of children.

Treatment Status of the Children

Parents were also asked to indicate if their child had ever received any of the following types of treatment:

Treatment type	Sample %
Any medication for a psychiatric or psychological disorder	8.1
Formal tutoring outside of school for school performance	4.1
Special education services of any type	9.4
Speech and language therapy	11.4
Occupational therapy	4.3
Physical therapy	3.0
Individual psychological counseling	9.4
Family psychological counseling	3.9
Group psychological therapy	0.9
Placement in an inpatient psychiatric unit	0.7
Attended a residential treatment school for children with psychological or psychiatric disorders	0.3
None of the treatments listed above	71.6

It is not possible to find comparable figures for the United States for all of these therapies, but a comparison on those for which figures are available suggests that these rates are reasonably similar to those found in other studies. For instance, one study using data from the National Ambulatory Medical Care Survey found a rate of psychotropic drug use of 8.3% for adolescents in 2000–2001 (Thomas, Conrad, Casler, & Goodman, 2006)—a figure that had more than doubled since 1996, and one very close to that found above for such drug use in the normative sample. Likewise, several studies found rates of 3.9–6.3% for children in the United States in 1996 (Olfson, Marcus, Weissman, & Jensen, 2002; Zito et al., 2003), a rate that also had more than doubled since 1987 (see Olfson et al., 2002). Given the results for the Thomas et al. study of teenagers over the subsequent term to 2001, this rate for children likely doubled again by the early 2000s (to at least 7–12%). Again, the expected rate is very similar to that found here.

The results for the factor analyses of the scale and construction of the individual subscales based on this normative sample are discussed in the next chapter.

CHAPTER 3

Factor Analysis, Scale Construction, and Item Frequencies

Factor analyses were used to uncover the underlying dimensions of SCT in the daily life activities of children and adolescents, as reported by their parents on the BSCTS-CA. This chapter discusses the results and how they were used to construct the final version and subscales of the BSCTS-CA. Thereafter, the frequencies with which the items were endorsed by the normative sample are presented and discussed.

Factor Analysis

As indicated in Chapter 2, the BSCTS-CA represents a set of items contained in a larger survey of ADHD, EF, and impairment items. It is important to show initially that the SCT items load on distinct dimensions of symptoms from those symptoms associated with ADHD, as has been found in numerous previous studies (see Chapter 1). This is to show that SCT is not simply a subtype or presentation of ADHD but is distinct from it in its symptom profile. The 14 items pertaining to SCT were analyzed by factor analysis along with the 18 items for ADHD from the DSM-IV (and 5, as all DSM-IV items were retained in the DSM-5) collected in the national survey. For the actual assessment of ADHD symptoms by a rating scale, I recommend the ADHD-5 Rating Scale by DuPaul and colleagues (DuPaul, Power, Anastopolos, & Reid, 2016).

Using the original and entire sample of 1,922 children, these 32 items were submitted to a principal components factor analysis (PCFA) using a varimax rotation. It is designed to maximize as many values in each column of the factor loading coefficient table as close to zero as possible. This approach is typically used in an attempt to reduce the degree of correlation among the items (variables). The results of the PCFA are shown in Table 3.1.

The first factor was labeled as the ADHD inattention dimension so commonly found in numerous prior studies of the ADHD symptom list. It contained 11 items, had an eigenvalue of 6.71 after rotation, and explained 20.9% of the variance after rotation. Nine of these items were from the DSM-5 inattention symptom list for ADHD, and the remaining two were from the 14 SCT items. These were (1) Slow to complete tasks, needs more time than others and (2) Lack initiative to complete work or their effort fades quickly after getting started. As a consequence, these symptoms are clearly not so much associated with SCT as with ADHD, and thus would not contribute to distinguishing these two conditions (ADHD vs. SCT) from each other. They were therefore eliminated from further consideration for inclusion in the BSCTS-CA.

The second factor had an eigenvalue of 6.35 after rotation, accounted for 19.8% of the variance after rotation, and contained the nine ADHD hyperactive–impulsive items, again consistent with numerous prior studies of the DSM symptom lists.

Factor 3 had an eigenvalue of 5.72 after rotation. It accounted for 17.9% of the variance after rotation and was comprised of 7 of the 14 SCT items. This dimension is labeled as Slow/Lethargic because of its two highest loading symptoms. The seven items having their highest loadings on this factor were:

1. Slow moving or sluggish
2. Lethargic, more tired than others or lacks energy
3. Has trouble staying alert or awake
4. Underactive compared to other children
5. Doesn't seem to understand or process questions or explanations as quickly as others
6. Seems drowsy, or has a sleepy appearance
7. Apathetic or withdrawn, seems less engaged in activities than others

The fourth factor had an eigenvalue of 3.16 and accounted for 9.9% of the variance after rotation. It clearly reflects the Daydreamy/Spacey/Mind Wandering dimension of SCT, so named here because of the three highest loading items, and identified previously by others (see Chapter 1). The five symptoms having their highest loadings on this factor were:

1. Prone to daydreaming
2. Spacey, his/her mind seems to be elsewhere
3. Gets lost in his/her own thoughts
4. Mentally foggy or easily confused
5. Stares a lot

The last two factors are clearly distinct from those of ADHD, are replicates of the dimensions found previously to comprise SCT, and are therefore retained to create the two subscales (Daydreamy/Spacey/Mind Wandering and Slow/Lethargic) of the BSCTS-CA. Important to note as well is that some of the items on the Slow/Lethargic dimension had nearly as high loadings on the Daydreamy/Spacey/

TABLE 3.1. Rotated Factor Loadings for BSCTS-CA Items Using PCFA with Varimax Rotation Based on Original Sample

Factor name/scale items	Factor number/item loading 1	2	3	4
Factor I: ADHD Inattention				
1. Fails to give close attention to details or makes careless mistakes in his/her work or other activities	**.754**	.244	.189	.120
2. Has difficulty sustaining his/her attention in tasks or fun activities	**.674**	.381	.218	.190
3. Doesn't listen when spoken to directly	**.604**	.426	.180	.180
4. Doesn't follow through on instructions and fails to finish work or chores	**.784**	.289	.159	.146
5. Has difficulty organizing tasks and activities	**.784**	.309	.168	.191
6. Avoids, dislikes, or is reluctant to engage in tasks that require sustained mental effort	**.759**	.287	.244	.112
7. Loses things necessary for tasks or activities	**.728**	.324	.187	.167
8. Easily distracted by extraneous stimuli or irrelevant thoughts	**.711**	.406	.142	.233
9. Forgetful in daily activities	**.710**	.310	.222	.274
Factor II: ADHD Hyperactivity–Impulsivity				
1. Fidgets with hands or feet or squirms in seat	.238	**.689**	.083	.247
2. Leaves his/her seat in classrooms or in other situations in which remaining seated is expected	.255	**.699**	.155	.260
3. Shifts around excessively or feels restless or hemmed in	.282	**.749**	.176	.229
4. Has difficulty engaging in leisure activities quietly (feels uncomfortable or is loud or noisy)	.333	**.695**	.270	.160
5. "On the go" or acts as if "driven by a motor" (or feels like he/she has to be busy or always doing something)	.245	**.748**	.041	.129
6. Talks excessively (in social situations)	.236	**.730**	.097	.085
7. Blurts out answers before questions have been completed; completes others' sentences or jumps the gun	.269	**.743**	.214	.100
8. Has difficulty waiting his/her turn	.312	**.737**	.174	.101
9. Interrupts or intrudes on others (butts into conversations or activities without permission or takes over what others are doing)	.305	**.743**	.152	.060
Factor IV: SCT Daydreamy				
1. Prone to daydreaming	.268	.191	.170	**.696**
2. Mentally foggy or easily confused	.248	.236	.525	**.534**
3. Stares a lot	.194	.274	.483	**.561**
4. Spacey; his/her mind seems to be elsewhere and not paying attention to what is going on around him/her	.307	.243	.409	**.665**
5. Gets lost in his/her thoughts	.250	.250	.386	**.613**

TABLE 3.1. *(continued)*

Factor name/scale items	Factor number/item loading			
	1	2	3	4
Factor III: SCT Sluggish				
1. Has trouble staying alert or awake	.191	.160	**.586**	.407
2. Lethargic, more tired than others, or lacks energy	.170	.135	**.833**	.156
3. Underactive compared to other children	.190	.111	**.832**	.054
4. Slow moving or sluggish	.172	.140	**.851**	.059
5. Doesn't seem to understand or process questions or explanations as quickly or as accurately as others	.401	.219	**.547**	.365
6. Seems drowsy or has a sleepy appearance	.135	.146	**.778**	.253
7. Apathetic or withdrawn; seems less engaged in activities than others	.215	.123	**.758**	.271
8. Slow to complete tasks, needs more time than others	**.515**	.241	.422	.391
9. Lacks initiative to complete work or his/her effort fades quickly after getting started	**.581**	.276	.428	.273

Note. $N = 1,922$ for the original sample. The highest loading of the item on a factor is indicated in **boldface type and underlining**.

Mind Wandering dimension, suggesting that these two dimensions share some overlapping variance with each other, as others have shown previously (Chapter 1).

Items measuring EF in daily life were also collected in this national survey. Given that ADHD has been previously shown to be associated with numerous deficits in EF in daily life activities (Barkley, 2012d) and may well be simply a proxy for a disorder of EF (Barkley, 2015b), it seemed important to the validity of these SCT factor dimensions to show that they are distinct from EF deficits as well. And so a PCFA using a varimax rotation was conducted using the 70 items of EF deficits from the Barkley Deficits in Executive Functioning Scale—Children and Adolescents (BDEFS-CA; Barkley, 2012d) and the 12 items from the SCT dimensions shown previously. The results revealed a seven-factor solution, with five of these factors being those previously identified for this EF rating scale (Barkley, 2012d). The remaining two factors were both distinct from these five EF dimensions as well as being identical in item composition to the preceding factor analysis of the SCT items in the context of the ADHD symptoms. Moreover, the content of these SCT items would not be considered to overlap with, or otherwise represent, commonly accepted descriptions of EF problems in daily life, as identified by others (Gioia, Isquith, Guy, & Kenworthy, 2000; Thorell & Nyberg, 2008). In short, the SCT items are not proxies for EF deficits in the daily life of children but are distinct factors from them. This finding also supports the position take earlier (Barkley, 2013) and in Chapter 1 that SCT does not appear to be a disorder of EF, as is ADHD, even though children having SCT may have some mildly elevated difficulties with WM (McBurnett et al., 2014) or organization and problem solving (Barkley, 2013). Such deficits are not similar to the substantial deficits children with ADHD have in those and other areas of EF.

Scale Construction

The 12 items of SCT discussed above and shown in Table 3.1 were used to create the subscales for the BSCTS-CA published here. All but two of the items were kept in their original sequence on the scale, just as they were presented to the normative sample during the survey. That original order is shown in the table as indicated by the number in front of each item. Because item arrangement or organization on a scale such as this has the potential to influence symptom endorsements by respondents (Mitchell, Knouse, Nelson-Gray, & Kwapil, 2009), items need to be arranged as close to their original sequence in the norming process as possible so as not to reduce the applicability of the norms for the final version of the scale. But two items (*Has trouble staying alert or awake; Gets lost in his/her thoughts*) had to be moved from that original sequence because the results of the PCFA (above) showed that the first item should actually be assigned to the Slow/Lethargic dimension and the second item to the Daydreamy/Spacey. By moving the item *Has trouble staying alert* to the position of being the first item on the Slow/Lethargic dimension within the scale, it follows right after the Daydreamy/Spacey symptoms with which it was originally placed. Likewise, the second item, *Gets lost in his/her thoughts,* is moved up the sequence to be the last item on the Daydreamy/Spacey subscale. Once this was done, the items were then renumbered sequentially to create the final version of the scale as it appears in the Appendix (not as it appears in Table 3.1). In sum, this method or organization of items on the scale retains the sequence and organization as near as possible to the manner in which it was given to the normative sample. It also permits ease of scoring because the examiner can simply sum the scores for the items in each section (subscale) to compute that subscale's score. The section or subscale total raw scores for the two SCT dimensions can be added together to create the SCT Total Score (see Chapter 8 for detailed scoring instructions). The examiner can then count the number of the 12 SCT items that were answered as "often" or "very often" (3 or 4) to also get an SCT Symptom Count score.

Frequency of Item Responses

It is clinically and scientifically informative to examine the percentage of parents in the normative sample (N= 1,800) who endorsed each of the responses for each item. This perspective gives an indication of how common or uncommon such symptoms of ADHD and SCT in daily life activities are likely to be in children and adolescents. This information can also be used to determine what frequency of occurrence for each item can be used to indicate that this item can be judged to be a "symptom" or actual deficit rather than a common occurrence in the population. For instance, if an item is answered by the vast majority of parents with an answer of "rarely" or "sometimes," then responses of "often" or "very often" can be considered to indicate a symptom of an attention disorder (ADHD or SCT) for a child. A symptom in this case would be a behavioral complaint that occurs at a frequency that is relatively low in the population and so may be indicative of a disorder. Whether it is or not so indicative, of course, is eventually a question of validity. That symptom should be examined against other forms of information so as to determine its correlates, particularly those dealing with impairment or functional ineffectiveness.

To gain some idea about how often parents endorse items describing ADHD and SCT symptoms in their child's daily life, the percentage of parents in the filtered normative sample (N = 1,800) that endorsed each of the possible answers to each item was computed. The results appear in Table 3.2. This is interesting information for child psychologists and others who may have an interest in knowing the proportion of the population that endorses particular types of ADHD or SCT symptoms at various relative frequencies. What this table clearly shows is that for the ADHD items, the vast majority of a general population sample of parents endorses most items at a frequency of either "never or rarely" or "sometimes." Answers of "often" or "very often" appeared to occur between 4.5 and 13% of the population, and in the majority of cases, less than 10% (though clearly there are a few exceptions). So if one wanted to identify a symptom of an attention disorder, it does not seem at all unreasonable to use an answer of "often" or "very often" to indicate the possibility of that item having symptom status. On average, less than 1 in 10 parents would endorse such answers about their child's behavior. The frequencies for endorsing similar answers reflective of a symptom ("often" or "very often") for the SCT items are even lower. Symptom endorsements ranged between just 2.4 and 6.1%, with the majority being endorsed under 4% of the time. One can see in this table that symptoms of ADHD occur more frequently in the population of U.S. children than do symptoms of SCT.

TABLE 3.2. Percent of the Normative Sample That Endorsed Each Possible Answer to Each Item on the BSCTS-CA

	Never or rarely	Sometimes	Often	Very often
Section 1: ADHD Inattention				
1. Fails to give close attention to details or makes careless mistakes in his/her work or other activities	51.7	35.8	8.9	3.5
2. Has difficulty sustaining his/her attention in tasks or fun activities	72.3	20.4	4.9	2.4
3. Doesn't listen when spoken to directly	63.9	28.7	4.6	2.8
4. Doesn't follow through on instructions and fails to finish work or chores	55.6	33.6	6.6	4.3
5. Has difficulty organizing tasks and activities	59.1	29.5	7.6	3.9
6. Avoids, dislikes, or is reluctant to engage in tasks that require sustained mental effort	63.3	26.7	6.1	3.8
7. Loses things necessary for tasks or activities	65.4	24.8	6.3	3.5
8. Easily distracted by extraneous stimuli or irrelevant thoughts	59.3	27.5	8.6	4.7
9. Forgetful in daily activities	63.7	27.2	5.5	3.7

(continued)

TABLE 3.2. *(continued)*

	Never or rarely	Sometimes	Often	Very often
Section 2: ADHD Hyperactivity–Impulsivity				
1. Fidgets with hands or feet or squirms in seat	67.3	22.4	6.6	3.7
2. Leaves his/her seat in classrooms or in other situations in which remaining seated is expected	83.1	12.2	2.6	2.1
3. Shifts around excessively or feels restless or hemmed in	77.0	16.3	3.8	2.8
4. Has difficulty engaging in leisure activities quietly (feels uncomfortable or is loud or noisy)	81.0	13.0	3.9	2.1
5. "On the go" or acts as if "driven by a motor" (or feels like he/she has to be busy or always doing something)	73.9	17.3	5.7	3.1
6. Talk excessively (in social situations)	65.0	23.7	7.1	4.2
7. Blurts out answers before questions have been completed, completes others' sentences, or jumps the gun	73.2	19.8	3.9	3.1
8. Has difficulty waiting his/her turn	70.8	22.0	4.4	2.8
9. Interrupts or intrudes on others (butts into conversations or activities without permission or takes over what others are doing)	64.5	25.6	5.9	4.1
Section 3: SCT Daydreamy				
1. Prone to daydreaming	66.6	27.4	4.1	2.0
2. Mentally foggy or easily confused	87.6	9.8	1.7	0.9
3. Stares a lot	87.7	9.1	2.1	1.1
4. Spacey; his/her mind seems to be elsewhere and not paying attention to what is going on around him/her	79.4	15.7	3.1	1.8
5. Gets lost in his/her thoughts	76.6	18.8	2.9	1.8
Section 4: SCT Sluggish				
1. Has trouble staying alert or awake	86.4	11.2	1.7	0.7
2. Lethargic, more tired than others, or lacks energy	85.5	11.7	1.7	1.1
3. Underactive compared to other children	83.2	12.2	3.2	1.4
4. Slow moving or sluggish	86.6	10.1	2.2	1.1
5. Doesn't seem to understand or process questions or explanations as quickly or as accurately as others	84.4	10.6	3.3	1.7
6. Seems drowsy, or has a sleepy appearance	89.6	8.1	1.6	0.8
7. Apathetic or withdrawn; seems less engaged in activities than others	85.8	10.9	2.2	1.1

Note. N = 1,800 for the normative sample.

The examiner should therefore focus not just on scoring the BSCTS-CA through simple summation of item responses, but should also inspect the scale for items pertaining to this attention disorder that were endorsed with responses of 3 (often) or 4 (very often). Those can be viewed as symptoms of the disorder (as endorsed by the parent completing the scale). This can provide another perspective on just how symptomatic a child may be for SCT, as assessed by the BSCTS-CA.

Creation of the Scores for the BSCTS-CA

As discussed earlier, using the item loadings shown in Table 3.1, items were grouped on the scale in sections representing their respective two dimensions for SCT, and the item sequences then renumbered sequentially. The sections of the scale were then organized in the same sequence they had been presented to the normative sample. There were five items on the SCT Daydreamy/Spacey factor (Section 1) and then seven items representing the Sluggish (Slow/Lethargic) SCT factor subscale (Section 2). After each list of SCT items, parents were asked to indicate at what age these symptoms first appeared, assuming they had answered that at least one symptom occurred often or more frequently (3 or 4). They were then asked whether or not (Yes/No) their child was impaired by those symptoms in any of four domains of major life activity: Home life with family, Social relations with other children, School, and Community activities (church, clubs, scouts, sports, etc.). All of these questions concerning symptoms, age of onset, and impairment comprise the BSCTS-CA. Items within each SCT factor subscale were then summed to create the raw score for that subscale, and the two SCT subscale scores were summed to create the SCT Total Score. One additional score was created that reflected the Total SCT Symptom Count across the two SCT sections. As noted above, a symptom was identified by an answer of 3 (often) or 4 (very often) to any of the items. Thus, four scores can be computed from the BSCTS-CA: (1) SCT Daydreamy Score, (2) SCT Sluggish Score, (3) SCT Total Score, and (4) SCT Symptom Count. These results are then plotted on the Profile scoring sheets for the child's age group and sex and for the answers to the age of onset and the domains of impairment questions.

The next chapter describes the relationship of these various BSCTS-CA scores to the demographic and other factors associated with the filtered normative sample of 1,800 parents. These issues pertain to the question of how best to present the norms provided in this manual for purposes of scoring the BSCTS-CA.

CHAPTER 4

Relationship of SCT Scores to Demographic Factors in the Normative Sample

This chapter describes the relationship of various demographic factors to the BSCTS-CA scores for the normative sample of 1,800 children.

Age

The age of the children was significantly and positively correlated with three of the four SCT scores: SCT Sluggish $r = .12$, $p < .001$; SCT Total Score = .09, $p < .001$, and SCT Symptom Count = .06, $p = .006$. (Note: Initial significance levels were set at $p \leq .01$ in all comparisons, given the large sample sizes in these analyses as well as the number of analyses to report in this chapter. Yet, one does not want to set the significance level too low and thus miss effects that may have importance in how the norms should be presented for scoring purposes in the Appendix.) These findings imply that both the severity and number of SCT symptoms increase slightly but significantly with age (which is in contrast to the modest decline evident in ADHD hyperactive–impulsive symptom severity noted in prior research—and in this survey). (See Chapter 1.)

However, correlation analyses may disguise nonlinear effects within such data. The relationships of age to the BSCTS-CA scores were therefore also analyzed using one-way analysis of variance (ANOVA) with the original 12 age groupings (6–17 years). The effect of age was significant again only for the SCT Sluggish score ($p = .001$). Pairwise comparisons (least significant difference) generally showed that 6- to 11-year-olds did not differ among themselves in these scores, but the 6- to 9-year-olds had significantly *lower* scores than those 12 years and older. Even when significant, such differences were less than 1 point on average. The results for the three SCT severity scores are displayed in Figure 4.1. The SCT Symptom Count is not shown, given its very low mean scores across age groups (0.2–0.6) and nonsignificance.

To summarize, age effects on the BSCTS-CA scores are small, are mainly nonlinear, are limited to the motor scores of SCT (Sluggish) and not the cognitive score (SCT Daydreamy), and primarily differ between the youngest and oldest six age groups (6- to 11-year-olds and 12- to 17-year-olds). These results mean that relatively large groupings of children based on age ranges can be done in presenting the norms without obscuring any potentially significant age differences that would have clinical significance on the motor score for this disorder. Age does not seem to matter, however, for the cognitive score for this disorder. The larger the age groupings that can be formed, the larger the sample sizes and the greater the likelihood that the norms so presented will be more reliable and representative of the U.S. population. Consequently, because of the significant age effects on the motor score, the norms in the Appendix are presented for the two groupings of 6- to 11-year-olds ($N = 902$) and 12- to 17-year-olds ($N = 898$), or six age levels collapsed within each grouping. This method is similar to what was done with other scales assessing symptoms of child psychopathology, such as the CBCL (Achenbach, 2001), and for much the same reasons.

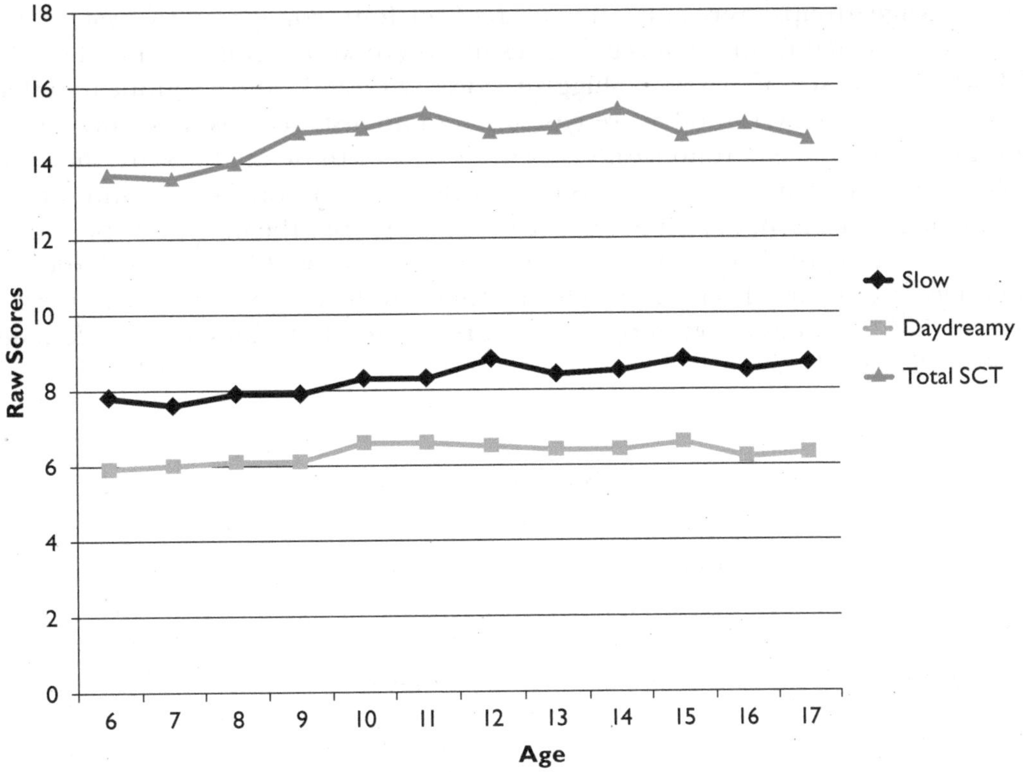

FIGURE 4.1. Raw scores of the 12 age groups for the three BSCTS-CA subscale scores for SCT ($N = 1{,}800$). Slow, Sluggish Score; Daydreamy, Daydreamy Score; Total SCT, SCT Total Score.

Sex Differences for Parents and Children

One-way ANOVAs were employed to compare the ratings of mothers and fathers ($N = 900$ each) on all four of the SCT scores. None of the comparisons were significant. Therefore, the sex of the parent completing the scale is not a significant factor in these normative data and thus of no concern in presenting the norms for scoring purposes in the Appendix.

A comparison of the 901 males with the 899 females from the normative sample ($N = 1{,}800$) indicated significant sex differences on just one of the four SCT scores: the Sluggish subscale score ($p = .004$). Boys were rated as having slightly but significantly more severe symptoms on this subscale than girls. The mean difference was quite small (0.4 points) and so of little clinical significance. So, for at least one of the SCT scores, it makes sense to present the norms in the Appendix for scoring purposes separately for each sex of child. Sex differences between children were also found for scales assessing symptoms of other dimensions of child psychopathology (Achenbach, 2001; Reynolds & Kamphaus, 2004). Therefore, norms presented separately for each sex on the BSCTS-CA Profile score sheets provided in the Appendix.

Using the normative sample, the next analyses examined if there was an interaction of child age with child sex on any of the BSCTS-CA scales. Two-way ANOVAs (sex × two age groups) were applied to each of the four scores from the BSCTS-CA scales. As expected from the foregoing results, there were significant main effects for both age and sex on the SCT Sluggish scores ($ps < .001$) and a significant effect for age only on the SCT Total Score ($p < .001$). In no instance was there any significant interaction of age group with sex. The results of those analyses are shown in Table 4.1. Consequently, because of the sex differences on some scores and the significant main effects for age on two of the four SCT scores, the norms are presented on the Profile score sheets separately for the two sexes within the two large age groupings of 6–11 and 12–17 years. This method produced separate norms for 451 males and 451 females between 6 and 11 years and for 450 males and 448 females between 12 and 17 years.

Ethnic Group

The next issue to address in considering how to best portray the norms for scoring purposes dealt with whether there exists any significant relationship of ethnic group to the BSCTS-CA scores. One-way ANOVAs revealed no significant effects of ethnic group on any of the SCT scores, nor did any comparisons even approach marginal significance ($p < .05$). This has also been the case for other rating scales of child psychopathology for use with parents (Achenbach, 2001; Reynolds & Kamphaus, 2004). Consequently, there seems to be little or no clinical value in displaying the norms for each ethnic group for scoring of the BSCTS-CA. All ethnic groups were therefore collapsed together in the portrayal of the norms on the scoring sheets in the Appendix.

TABLE 4.1. Means and Standard Deviations for the BSCTS-CA Scores for Each Sex within Each of the Two Age Groups Used to Create the SCT Profiles in the Appendix

	Age groups × sex									
	6–11 years				12–17 years					
	Males		Females		Males		Females			
	Mean	*SD*	Mean	*SD*	Mean	*SD*	Mean	*SD*	*F*	*p*
SCT Daydreamy Score	6.2	2.4	6.2	2.3	6.5	2.5	6.3	2.2	A = 2.49 S = 2.44 A × S = 0.89	NS NS NS
SCT Sluggish Score	8.0	2.6	7.9	2.6	9.0	3.6	8.3	2.8	A = 22.89 S = 8.49 A × S = 3.75	<.001 .004 NS
SCT Total Score	14.3	4.7	14.1	4.6	15.5	5.8	14.6	4.6	A = 12.87 S = 6.10 A × S = 2.54	<.001 NS NS
SCT Symptom Count Score	0.4	1.4	0.3	1.4	0.7	2.0	0.4	1.4	A = 4.87 S = 5.24 A × S = 2.60	NS NS NS

Note. F, results for the *F*-test from the analysis of variance; A, main effect for age group; S, main effect for sex; A × S, interaction of age group × sex; *p*, probability value for each of the *F*-tests if ≤.01; NS, not significant.

Parent Education and Household Income

Correlations were computed between the educational level of the respondent parents in the normative sample and all four of the BSCTS-CA scores. All four SCT scores were statistically significant but trivially related to parent educational level in a negative way. The lower the education level the greater the symptoms of SCT reported in the children. The correlations were SCT Sluggish $r = -.08$; SCT Daydreamy = –.08; SCT Total Score = –.09; and SCT Symptom Count = –.08; all *p*s < .001.

The same results were evident for the correlations between household income level and the four scores from the BSCTS-CA. In this case, all of the correlations reached significance. The correlations ranged from only –.08 to –.12 (all *p*s < .001). Parents with less household income reported slightly higher scores on all BSCTS-CA scores. But, again, the shared variance here is 1% or less and of little consequence for the reporting of the normative results. The same low but significant relationships between executive functioning scores and parent education and income have been reported for other parent rating scales of EF (Gioia et al., 2000). These relationships are likely significant owing to the large sample size use here (N = 1,800). If anything, such findings may be modest evidence of validity, in that greater difficulties with SCT in children, just as with symptoms of child psychopathology, would be expected to be somewhat greater in the lowest educational and income groups. As a result, the educational and income levels were collapsed together for portrayal of the norms.

Geographic Region

Potential differences in the scores from the scale with regard to geographic regions were evaluated using one-way ANOVA comparing the four major regions of the United States using the normative sample (N = 1,800). There were no significant differences for any of the scores, nor did any of the scores even approach marginal significance. It is therefore reasonable to collapse the geographic regions together for purposes of displaying the normative information on this sample.

Conclusions

In view of the above findings and discussion, four separate BSCTS-CA Profile score sheets are provided in the Appendix, containing the various raw scores and their associated percentiles for males ages 6–11 (N = 451), males ages 12–17 (N = 450), females ages 6–11 (N = 451), and females ages 12–17 (N = 448).

CHAPTER 5

Reliability

This brief chapter presents the information that is available concerning the various forms of reliability for the BSCTS-CA. Obviously, more research on these and other psychometric characteristics of the scale is to be encouraged. However, the information that is available indicates that the reliabilities of the scale scores are satisfactory and support the use of the BSCTS-CA in clinical practice and research when the assessment of parental reports concerning the two attention disorders in the daily life activities of their children is of interest.

Subscale Relationships

As indicated by the factor analysis reported earlier, ratings of SCT in daily life activities, just like those for ADHD, each appear to be comprised of two dimensions, one for cognitive (for SCT, Daydreamy; for ADHD, Inattention) and the other for motoric or behavioral (for SCT, Sluggish; for ADHD, Hyperactive–Impulsive). We should therefore not be surprised to find that the BSCTS-CA scales created from these SCT dimensions are likewise interrelated within each disorder more than with dimensions of the other disorder, and so are partially separable. In one sense, this separable aspect reflects a form of internal consistency in the scale. Are the subscales of SCT sufficiently related to each other so as to be clustered under the same construct or condition?

The relationships among the scales were evaluated using Pearson product–moment correlations using the entire original sample of 1,922 participants. The results, shown in Table 5.1, clearly indicate that the ADHD items in the survey are far more highly related to each other than to the subscale scores for SCT, and vice versa. Even so, scores for one disorder are significantly related to the scores for

TABLE 5.1. Comparison of Initial and Retesting Sample Results on the BSCTS-CA Long and Short Form Scores

	Initial		Retesting		Mean		
	Mean	*SD*	Mean	*SD*	diff.	*t*	*p*
SCT Daydreamy Score	6.3	2.9	6.4	2.7	<0.1	−0.48	NS
SCT Sluggish Score	8.3	3.6	8.2	3.2	<0.1	0.31	NS
SCT Total Score	14.6	6.3	14.6	5.6	<0.1	−0.06	NS
ADHD Inattention Score	13.9	6.0	14.0	6.4	<0.1	−0.30	NS
ADHD Hyperactivity–Impulsivity Score	12.4	5.3	13.2	6.6	0.7	−1.92	NS
ADHD Total Score	26.3	10.6	27.2	12.3	0.9	−1.29	NS

Note. $N = 86$. Mean diff., differences in the initial and retesting means; *t*, results for the paired-samples *t*-test; *p*, probability value for the *t*-test if ≤.01; NS, not significant.

the other, in part due to the large sample size used in computing these correlations. Squaring these correlations indicates the degree of variance shared between a score for one disorder, such as ADHD, with the score for the other disorder, SCT. For instance, ADHD Inattention shares 42% of its variance with that of SCT Daydreamy and 31% of its variance with SCT Sluggish. Hence, although ADHD is distinct from SCT, there is clearly some overlap between the cognitive dimensions of these two attention disorders. In contrast, ADHD Hyperactivity–Impulsivity shares about 35% of its variance with the SCT Daydreamy dimension and just 22% of its variance with the SCT Sluggish dimension. In all of these instances, the majority of the variance in each dimension is *not* shared with the variance in each dimension of the other disorder. Such overlap does suggest that their may be some comorbidity between these two conditions, perhaps owing to some shared etiological factor, such as was found in genetic heritability by Moruzzi et al. (2014), yet there is also unique unshared genetic variance between the disorders.

Given that the two dimensions within each disorder are quite highly correlated with each other, it would seem important to remove that overlap when examining their relationships to the dimensions of the other disorder, as such shared relationships within a disorder could inflate the association with the dimensions of the other. To that effect, partial correlations were used to examine the association of ADHD Inattention with the two SCT scores, removing ADHD Hyperactivity–Impulsivity from this association. The correlations drop to $r = .40$ for the SCT Daydreamy Score and to $r = .36$ for the SCT Sluggish dimension when this is done, indicating that ADHD Inattention now shares just 16% and 13% of its variance with these respective SCT dimensions, once the overlap or contamination of ADHD Inattention with Hyperacivity–Impulsivity is statistically removed. Likewise, the relationship of ADHD Hyperactivity–Impulsivity falls to $r = .23$ (5% shared variance) with the SCT Daydreamy dimension, and to $r = .11$ (1% shared variance) with the Sluggish dimension when the overlap with ADHD Inattention is statistically removed. Yet the relationship between the two SCT dimensions remains moderate to high in magnitude (*r*s = .66 and .61) even after ADHD Inattention and

Hyperactivity–Impulsivity are statistically removed from those associations (sharing 36%+ of their variance). The respective correlations between the two ADHD dimensions (*r*s = .55 and .63; 30 and 40% shared variance, respectively) also remain moderate or greater in magnitude, even after removing the SCT Daydreamy and Sluggish scores, respectively, from these relationships. This finding makes it much clearer that the two dimensions of SCT share far more variance with each other, even after controlling for overlap with ADHD, than do the dimensions of each disorder with those of the other disorder. In short, SCT and ADHD, although overlapping, are quite distinct from each other.

Internal Consistency

The internal consistency (Chronbach's alpha) of each of the three SCT subscale scores was computed based on the entire sample of 1,922 and found to be quite satisfactory: SCT Daydreamy = .872, SCT Sluggish = .912, and SCT Total Score = .934. All *F*-tests were significant at $p < .001$. Given that the symptom count score is made up of these same items, it was not necessary to compute those internal consistencies. Such results are quite comparable to other rating scales of psychopathology in children (Achenbach, 2001; Reynolds & Kamphaus, 2004) and to the adult and child versions of the ADHD-5 Rating Scale (Barkley, 2011a; DuPaul et al., 2016). Thus, the internal consistency of the subscales is quite satisfactory.

Test–Retest Reliability

Test–retest reliability reflects the temporal consistency of a measure, particularly over shorter time intervals that are unlikely to be substantially impacted by developmental factors in children. It was assessed by having a subset of the original sample participants complete the scale on a second occasion, 3–5 weeks after initially completing the scale. A total of 86 parents completed the scale a second time, with at least five children for each age level from 6 to 17 years. There were 45 boys and 41 girls in this sample. The breakdown for the sex of the parent was 36 males and 50 females. These parents were randomly chosen by Knowledge Networks within each age group and sex and invited to return to the website to complete the scale for a second time.

The Pearson product–moment correlations between the first and second administrations were: SCT Daydreamy Score = .79 ($p < .001$), SCT Sluggish Score = .82 ($p < .001$), and SCT Total Score = .84 ($p < .001$). These results are quite satisfactory and indicate a reasonable level of test–retest reliability over this 3- to 5-week period. They are also relatively comparable to the test–retest reliability correlations found for other rating scales of psychopathology for children (Achenbach, 2001; Reynolds & Kamphaus, 2004).

The actual scores from the initial testing and retesting administrations were then compared using a paired-samples *t*-test. The results, shown in Table 5.1, indicated that none of the three subscale scores changed significantly across this 3- to

5-week test–retest interval. Again, because symptom counts are comprised of these same items, that score was not analyzed here.

Conclusions

This brief chapter demonstrates that the BSCTS-CA has quite satisfactory levels of various forms of internal as well as cross-temporal consistency (test–retest reliability). The findings are sufficient to support the use of the BSCTS-CA as a reliable measure of SCT in the daily life activities of children.

CHAPTER 6

Validity

This chapter presents the information that is available concerning several important forms of validity regarding the scores from the BSCTS-CA. As with the information on reliability in the previous chapter, more research on these forms of validity and other psychometric characteristics of the scale is to be welcomed. Nevertheless, the information currently available and discussed in this chapter indicates that the validity of the scale is quite reasonable or acceptable. Such information supports the use of the BSCTS-CA in clinical practice and research when the assessment of parental reports concerning attention disorders in the daily life activities of their children is of interest.

The term "validity" typically refers to the correctness, accuracy, or truth of an assertion or conclusion as judged against the empirical evidence (Bryant, 2000). In this instance of measurement development, it refers to the extent to which the rating scale measures what it claims to assess. To what extent is the BSCTS-CA measuring attention deficits in the daily life activities of children? And to what degree is it useful in doing so? Much of the work of validating the BSCTS-CA comes from the national survey reported in this manual. However, given the strong similarity to, if not the identical nature of, the items on this scale to other rating scales of SCT used in previous studies and discussed in Chapter 1, the results of those studies can also be taken as indirect evidence of the validity of BSCTS-CA. The evidence that is currently available regarding the validity of this exact scale is satisfactory and supports the use of this scale as a measure of SCT in daily life-activity-related deficits in children 6–17 years.

Construct and Convergent Validity

As noted by others, construct validity starts with an explicit definition of the construct that a measure is intended to assess (Bryant, 2000; Cook & Campbell, 1979).

Otherwise, one cannot determine if the measure is accurately or correctly sampling from, and hence evaluating, the conceptual (semantic) domain of this construct. Because this scale uses most of the items identified in prior studies as comprising the condition of SCT (see Chapter 1), it also has acceptable face validity as a measure of SCT symptoms reported by parents.

A related form of validity to construct validity is convergent validity. Do various measures of the same construct converge or agree? The BSCTS-CA certainly would be expected to show high correlations with other rating scales using most or all of these 12 SCT symptoms (see Chapter 1). So although the BSCTS-CA has not been evaluated for its correlation with other comparable measures of SCT, given the existing evidence, it would undoubtedly do so because its item content is nearly identical to other such scales used in research on SCT.

Evidence from Factor Analyses

Some evidence for how well the BSCTS-CA captures SCT symptom dimensions became evident in the research conducted over the past decade with similar or identical rating scales and the results of factor or dimensional analyses of those scales (see Chapter 1). Their results were virtually identical to those discussed in Chapter 3 of this manual, which set forth the results of the factor analysis of the BSCTS-CA. In short, the items on the present scale formed the same dimensions as those found in prior research using these same items. This identicalness provides corroboration of the content or conceptual validity of the scale.

Divergent or Discriminant Validity

We turn now to evidence of divergent or discriminant validity. As Bryant (2000) has explained, this term refers to evidence that the constructs of SCT, as evaluated by the BSCTS-CA, differ from each other and from other psychological constructs that the instrument is not intended to evaluate or measure. It is the opposite of convergent validity, in which measures of the same construct ought to converge on or correlate with one another, as above.

Relationship to Intelligence (IQ)

SCT, like ADHD, is not considered to be identical to the construct of intelligence or IQ. Given how it is conceptualized, one might expect a modest relationship between SCT, given that its symptoms might adversely impact performance on an IQ test, such as on items involving organization and WM. But the field of psychology generally treats IQ and attention disorders as distinct concepts. It is therefore important to show that the content of the BSCTS-CA is largely not contaminated with measurements of intelligence. No evidence currently exists on the relationship of the present parent form of the BSCTS-CA to measures of IQ. But prior findings with SCT scales that contained items highly similar or even identical to those of the BSCTS-CA are relevant. As noted in Chapter 1, past research has found that ratings are low and inconsistently related to IQ (*r*s = –.15 to +.25; Becker, Leopold, et al., 2016). Essentially, ratings of SCT share less than 6% of their variance with IQ. Obviously, ratings of SCT are not proxies for, nor do they significantly overlap with measures of, IQ, and hence are a distinct construct from IQ.

Relationship to EF

The relationship of ADHD ratings to measures of EF continues to be controversial and is highly related to the type of measures used to assess the construct of EF (Barkley, 2012b, 2012d). Groups selected for having elevated symptoms of ADHD often manifest differences on a number of EF tests from typical groups (Frazier et al., 2004; Hervey et al., 2004; Willcutt, 2015; Willcutt et al., 2005), usually in inhibition, attention, and WM, and to a lesser extent and less consistently in planning and problem solving. Yet when examined at the individual level, only 12–50% (and typically less than 35%) of such cases show deficient performance on EF tests (Barkley, 2012d, 2015b; Biederman et al., 2008; Willcutt, 2015; Willcutt et al., 2005). This fact has led some reviewers to argue that ADHD is not simply a disorder of EF (Willcutt, 2015) and that other or multiple pathway theories of the disorder are needed. However, on ratings of EF in daily life, groups comprised of people with elevated ADHD symptom ratings often show far more substantial and widespread deficits, and these deficits afflict the vast majority of those having ADHD (Barkley, 2011c, 2012d; Barkley & Fischer, 2011; Barkley & Murphy, 2010). Moreover, the high correlations between ratings of ADHD and ratings of EF indicate that at least 40–70%+ of the variance in either measure is shared with the other measure (especially ADHD Inattention). This finding suggests that ADHD and EF may represent the same construct (Barkley, 2011c, 2012d). Such a gross disparity in the results between EF tests and EF ratings in their relationship to ADHD ratings arises, in large part, because there is no significant correlation between these two forms of measuring EF (Toplak, West, & Stanovich, 2013). Given that ratings of EF are more predictive of impairments in major domains of daily life activities than are EF tests (Barkley & Fischer, 2011; Barkley & Murphy, 2010), the evidence from ratings of EF would seem to be the more valid index of EF in those having ADHD.

Using the same U.S. normative sample, as described here, and the ADHD symptom item ratings in the national survey, I (Barkley, 2013) reported these regression analyses. Those results showed that ratings of ADHD contributed the following amounts of variance to the five dimensions of EF contained on the BDEFS-CA. For ADHD Inattention, the variance predicted was 63% in EF ratings of Self-Management to Time, 55% to Self-Organization and Problem Solving, 59% to Self-Restraint (inhibition), 77% to Self-Motivation, and 49% to Self-Regulation of Emotion. For ADHD Hyperactivity–Impulsivity, the variances contributed to EF ratings were <1% to Self-Management to Time, <1% to Self-Organization and Problem Solving, 6% to Self-Restraint, <1% to Self-Motivation, and 6% to Self-Regulation of Emotion. Clearly, it is ADHD Inattention that has the greatest overlap with EF ratings and thus can be viewed as nearly synonymous with it, whereas ADHD Hyperactivity–Impulsivity is far less related to EF in daily life and, as expected, related more to the EF dimensions involving inhibition, albeit to a very low extent. Thus, ADHD (especially its inattention symptoms) can be viewed as a form of EF deficit disorder (EFDD) when ratings of both are used, whereas ADHD

Hyperactive–Impulsive symptoms principally reflect motor and verbal hyperactivity (and not behavioral inhibition or self-restraint to any great extent).

This is not the case for ratings of SCT as measured on the BSCTS-CA. As shown in Chapter 3, factor analysis of SCT ratings combined with EF ratings show that the two symptom dimensions of SCT emerge as distinct from those of EF. Also, prior research on EF deficits in those having SCT, whether using tests or ratings, finds far less evidence of EF deficits linked to SCT and, when found, are far milder in degree (Becker, Leopold, et al., 2016). Table 6.1 shows the results of the regression analyses conducted on this U.S. sample (Barkley, 2013). The SCT Daydreamy symptoms contributed the following amounts of variance to the EF dimensions: 0% to Self-Management to Time, <1% to Self-Organization and Problem Solving, <1% to Self-Restraint, <1% to Self-Motivation, and nothing to Self-Regulation of Emotion.

TABLE 6.1. Regression Analyses of the ADHD and SCT Symptom Dimensions onto the Summary Scores from the BDEFS-CA

Rating scale/symptom predictors	Beta	*R*	R^2	$R^2\Delta$	*F*	*p*
BDEFS-CA Self-Management to Time						
ADHD Inattention Symptoms	.763	.796	.634	.634	3326.81	<.001
ADHD Hyperactive–Impulsive Symptoms	.045	.797	.635	.001	1669.59	<.001
BDEFS-CA Self-Organization and Problem Solving						
ADHD Inattention Symptoms	.489	.744	.553	.553	2379.67	<.001
SCT Sluggish Symptoms	.153	.770	.593	.039	1396.26	<.001
SCT Daydreaming Symptoms	.136	.776	.602	.009	967.78	<.001
ADHD Hyperactive–Impulsive Symptoms	.112	.780	.608	.006	742.66	<.001
BDEFS-CA Self-Restraint						
ADHD Inattention Symptoms	.540	.771	.595	.595	2820.39	<.001
ADHD Hyperactive–Impulsive Symptoms	.365	.809	.654	.059	1811.30	<.001
SCT Daydreaming Symptoms	–.052	.809	.655	.001	1214.73	<.001
BDEFS-CA Self-Motivation						
ADHD Inattention Symptoms	.830	.878	.771	.771	6465.51	<.001
SCT Sluggish Symptoms	.099	.880	.774	.003	3283.48	<.001
SCT Daydreams Symptoms	–.072	.880	.775	.001	2203.96	<.001
ADHD Hyperactive–Impulsive Symptoms	.054	.881	.776	.001	1664.61	<.001
BDEFS-CA Self-Regulation of Emotion						
ADHD Inattention Symptoms	.408	.698	.487	.487	1823.25	<.001
ADHD Hyperactive–Impulsive Symptoms	.337	.738	.545	.058	1147.39	<.001
SCT Sluggish Symptoms	.082	.741	.549	.005	778.67	<.001

Note. Analyses are linear multiple regression with stepwise entry. Beta, standardized beta coefficient from the final model; *R*, regression coefficient; R^2, percent of explained variance accounted for by all variables at this step; $R^2\Delta$ (change), percent of explained variance accounted for by this variable added at this step; *F*, *F* to change results; *p*, probability value for the *F*-test. Adapted from Barkley (2013). Copyright © Taylor & Francis. Adapted by permission.

Likewise, the SCT Sluggish dimension contributed little if anything to these same five EF dimensions: nothing to Self-Management to Time, 4% to Self-Organization and Problem Solving, nothing to Self-Restraint, <1% to Self-Motivation, and <1% to Self-Regulation of Emotion. Such evidence supports the position that the constructs underlying SCT do not overlap significantly with the constructs of EF, at least in children, and so ratings of SCT, as measured on the BSCTS-CA, have substantial divergent validity from those of EF. That is not the case for ADHD (especially the inattention dimension), which shares substantial overlap with components of EF in daily life.

Nevertheless, it should be noted that by adulthood, self-ratings of SCT do appear to make a significant contribution to some EF components. For instance, SCT ratings contribute 66% of the variance and ADHD Inattention just 4% of the variance to Self-Organization and Problem Solving (Barkley, 2012a). But ADHD Inattention contributes 54% of the variance to Time Management, whereas SCT contributes just 5% of the variance (Barkley, 2012a). ADHD Hyperactive–Impulsive symptoms make no significant contribution to either EF scale. For the EF component of Self-Restraint (inhibition), the contributions include 46% for SCT, 8% for ADHD Hyperactive–Impulsive, and 2% for ADHD Inattention. For the EF component of Self-Motivation, the findings were 49% for ADHD Inattention, 3% for SCT, and <1% for ADHD Hyperactive–Impulsive. For the Self-Regulation of Emotion component of EF, the results were 44% for SCT, 8% for ADHD Hyperactive–Impulsive, and 1% for ADHD Inattention. For whatever reason, by adulthood the influence of SCT symptoms makes a far greater and majority contribution to the EF components of Self-Organization, Self-Restraint (or self-discipline), and Self-Regulation of Emotions compared to ADHD symptoms. Why this is the case is not clear, but it does help to understand why SCT was found to be so much more impairing in adult functioning in various major domains of life activities, such as work and education, than was the case for children (Barkley, 2012a, 2013). Even so, in this manual we are concerned with the relationships of ADHD and SCT to EF in children, and in that age range, we find little association of SCT with these same EF components.

Relationship to Academic Achievement Tests

Both ADHD and SCT are conceptualized as distinctly different constructs from those measured by academic achievement tests. Those tests essentially reflect the level of knowledge of particular academic subjects someone possesses or basic academic achievement skills, such as reading, math, and spelling. This is not to say that ADHD and SCT are unimportant to the acquisition of academic knowledge and achievement skills, only that they are not intended to represent that end state of acquired academic skill and information. As discussed in Chapter 1 and elsewhere (Becker, Leopold, et al., 2016; DuPaul & Langberg, 2015), both ADHD and SCT are linked to substantial impairment in performance in educational settings. There are many reasons both disorders would cause such problems—particularly their adverse impact on behavior and availability for learning in such settings—apart from their relationship to actual academic achievement tests and academic skills.

As discussed in Chapter 1, and in the meta-analysis by Becker, Leopold, et al. (2016), SCT shows a very inconsistent and weak relationship to measures of academic achievement. A few studies suggest that the relationship may be somewhat greater with math achievement than reading or spelling. But generally the relationship is small, which suggests that SCT, as a construct, is quite divergent from academic achievement skills. ADHD has a somewhat stronger relationship to measures of academic achievement (DuPaul & Langberg, 2015; Frazier et al., 2004; Hervey et al., 2004). People with ADHD perform more poorly on academic achievement tests, on average, beginning in the early childhood years and continuing into adulthood (Barkley, Murphy, & Fischer, 2008; DuPaul & Langberg, 2015), scoring on average about half to three-quarters of a standard deviation (the effect size) below typical people, with reading being more affected than math achievement. In part, this finding is related to the considerable comorbidity of LDs with ADHD (30–45%; DuPaul & Langberg, 2015), but may be evident even in those who do not manifest such comorbidity. Nevertheless, correlations between ADHD ratings and academic achievement are small to moderate in size, suggest a shared variance of less than 25%, and thus appear to be divergent constructs. Therefore, one would expect that ratings of SCT, as collected by the BSCTS-CA, would have such small-to-moderate relationships with measures of academic achievement skills, yet not be considered to evaluate the same constructs.

Criterion Validity: Degree of SCT Symptoms in Other Disorders

Problems with inattention are common across many developmental and psychiatric disorders. Thus, one would expect that many psychiatric disorders in children would be associated with higher ratings on the SCT dimensions assessed on the BSCTS-CA. Granted, some of this relationship arises due to the comorbidity between SCT and ADHD and so between ADHD and these other disorders, such as that with LDs noted above, or even more often with disruptive disorders such as ODD and conduct disorder (Angold et al., 1999). There is a plethora of research showing that many child psychiatric and developmental disorders have higher scores on ADHD ratings than do typical children, far too numerous to review here. For instance, children with both speech sound disorders and specific language impairments may have significantly greater likelihood of having ADHD, ranging from 16 to 66% (McGrath et al., 2008), and thus would show elevated ratings of such.

There is substantially less research on this issue concerning SCT ratings. To help address that dearth of information, here I employ the national U.S. survey described in this manual. In that survey, parents reported whether their child had ever received a professional diagnosis of any of 17 different psychiatric or developmental disorders. These diagnoses are listed in Table 6.2; this table also shows the extent of elevated ratings on SCT dimensions from the BSCTS-CA for each of those 17 diagnoses. Given that there is a small to moderate association of ADHD with SCT (particularly for ADHD Inattention), the mean scores for each of these ratings within the diagnostic groups has had the relationship to the other attention disorder statistically removed (covaried) prior to the statistical analysis of any group differences between the disordered and nondisordered groups. Multivariate analyses of variance were used to evaluate the differences between each disordered and nondisordered (control) group of children on the two ADHD symptom dimensions collected in the survey, controlling for total SCT ratings. If significant (at $p <$ .01), then the individual ANOVA results for each ADHD subscale were examined for significance, which was set at $p < .05$. Then the same procedure was followed in comparing the disordered to nondisordered groups on the two SCT subscales from the BSCTS-CA, controlling for total ADHD symptoms (covariate). In short, the SCT ratings were statistically removed from all results for the ADHD dimensions, and the ADHD ratings were removed from all results for the SCT dimensions.

Most of the disorders listed in Table 6.2 showed significantly elevated ratings of both ADHD and SCT dimensions even after controlling for the overlap between these two attention disorders. Although such findings of elevated rates of ADHD symptoms in most other disorders are not especially new, given elevated rates of comorbidity of ADHD with these other disorders (Angold et al., 1999; Brown, 2009), the findings that high SCT symptoms are associated with these disorders *independent* of the overlap of SCT with ADHD, are new, supporting the validity of both SCT as a disorder and the BSCTS-CA scores. Specifically, ADHD Inattention symptoms were significantly elevated, compared to control participants, in most disorders; the exceptions included children with physical disability, tic disorders, seizure disorder, conduct disorder, depression, and bipolar disorder. Likewise, nearly all of the disorders in Table 6.2 also showed elevated levels of ADHD Hyperactive symptoms, excepting for children with physical disability, math disorders, seizure disorder, and depression. The fact that most disorders have elevated ratings of ADHD symptoms after controlling for the overlap with SCT is, as noted above, very consistent with the significant comorbidity of ADHD with these other disorders, and vice versa (Angold et al., 1999; Brown, 2009; Pliszka, 2015). The lack of elevated symptoms of either ADHD symptom dimension in children diagnosed with depression seems puzzling at first, given that depression has been found to coexist with ADHD in some studies, though not all (Pliszka, 2015). However, recall that the SCT ratings were removed from these findings and that earlier research (see Chapter 1) suggested that SCT has a far stronger relationship to depression than does ADHD. Indeed, some research suggested that the overlap of SCT with ADHD might even account for the apparent relationship of ADHD to depression. The findings here are consistent with that idea. The lack of any significant elevation in ADHD Inattention for children with conduct disorder, even though they had elevated ADHD Hyperactivity–Impulsivity symptoms, is not so surprising, given past research showing that it is the latter dimension of ADHD that is most closely aligned with antisocial behavior (Barkley et al., 2008). It is possible that the lack of significant results for children with physical disability, tic disorders, and seizure disorder may be due to the very small prevalence and hence sample sizes for those disorders in this U.S. population sample.

Noteworthy as well is that the patterns for significantly elevated SCT symptoms were not the same as those for ADHD symptoms across the disorders in Table 6.2. Significantly elevated symptoms of SCT were evident in many disorders, even after controlling for ADHD symptoms. But elevated SCT symptoms were not evident in the following disorders: physically disabled, reading disorder, spelling disorder, other academic disorders, and tic disorders. In contrast, ADHD symptoms *were* elevated in cases having reading, spelling, and other academic disorders. The Daydreamy dimension of SCT was elevated in children diagnosed with writing, sei-

TABLE 6.2. Adjusted (Marginal) Means, Standard Errors, and Effect Sizes for the ADHD Symptom Scores and the SCT Subscale Scores from the BSCTS-CA

	ADHD Scores				SCT Scores				
	IN		HI		Daydreamy		Sluggish		
Diagnostic groups	Mean	*SE*	Mean	*SE*	Mean	*SE*	Mean	*SE*	*n*
Physical disability	13.9	1.8	11.7	1.7	7.1	0.7	10.1	1.0	6
Controls	13.7	0.1	12.4	0.1	6.3	<0.1	8.3	<0.1	1,916
p (if significant)	NS		NS		NS		NS		
ES (*d*)	0.02		−0.11		0.19		0.30		
Language delay	15.5	0.5	13.5	0.4	6.9	0.2	9.3	0.2	96
Controls	13.6	0.1	12.4	0.1	6.3	<0.1	8.2	<0.1	1,826
p	<.001		.017		<.001		<.001		
ES (*d*)	0.26		0.17		0.19		0.27		
Motor delay	17.0	0.6	14.2	0.5	7.1	0.2	9.3	0.3	63
Controls	13.6	0.1	12.4	0.1	6.3	<0.1	8.2	<0.1	1,859
p	<.001		.001		<.001		.001		
ES (*d*)	0.47		0.29		0.25		0.27		
Reading disorder	17.8	0.5	14.4	0.5	6.4	0.2	8.5	0.3	77
Controls	13.5	0.1	12.3	0.1	6.3	<0.1	8.3	<0.1	1,845
p	<.001		<.001		NS		NS		
ES (*d*)	0.61		0.32		0.03		0.05		
Math disorder	17.5	0.7	13.0	0.6	7.1	0.3	9.3	0.4	44
Controls	13.6	0.1	12.4	0.1	6.3	<0.1	8.3	<0.1	1,878
p	<.001		NS		.003		.005		
ES (*d*)	0.57		0.09		0.27		0.24		
Spelling disorder	17.7	0.7	13.9	0.6	6.7	0.3	8.7	0.4	45
Controls	13.6	0.1	12.4	0.1	6.3	<0.1	8.3	<0.1	1,877
p	<.001		.019		NS		NS		
ES (*d*)	0.60		0.24		0.15		0.12		
Writing disorder	18.3	0.7	14.4	0.7	7.2	0.3	9.0	0.4	43
Controls	13.6	0.1	12.4	0.1	6.3	<0.1	8.3	<0.1	1,879
p	<.001		.003		<.001		NS		
ES (*d*)	0.66		0.32		0.29		0.19		
Other academic disorders	17.8	0.8	14.2	0.7	7.1	0.3	9.0	0.4	33
Controls	13.6	0.1	12.4	0.1	6.3	<0.1	8.3	<0.1	1,889
p	<.001		.015		NS		NS		
ES (*d*)	0.62		0.32		0.24		0.16		

TABLE 6.2. *(continued)*

	ADHD Scores				SCT Scores				
	IN		HI		Daydreamy		Sluggish		
Diagnostic groups	Mean	*SE*	Mean	*SE*	Mean	*SE*	Mean	*SE*	*n*
General developmental delay	17.5	1.0	14.9	0.9	8.5	0.4	11.1	0.5	22
Controls	13.6	0.1	12.4	0.1	6.3	<0.1	8.3	<0.1	1,900
p	<.001		.01		<.001		<.001		
ES (*d*)	0.51		0.34		0.61		0.60		
Tics/Tourette syndrome	15.7	1.3	16.6	1.3	6.1	0.5	9.7	0.7	11
Controls	13.6	0.1	12.4	0.1	6.3	<0.1	8.3	<0.1	1,911
p	NS		.001		NS		NS		
ES (*d*)	0.30		0.65		−0.06		0.30		
Seizure disorder	14.9	1.2	11.7	1.1	7.7	0.5	8.7	0.6	12
Controls	13.6	0.1	12.4	0.1	6.3	<0.1	8.3	<0.1	1,908
p	NS		NS		.002		NS		
ES (*d*)	0.18		−0.12		0.52		0.14		
ADHD	19.3	0.3	17.9	0.3	6.1	0.1	7.6	0.2	173
Controls	13.1	0.1	11.9	0.1	6.3	<0.1	8.3	<0.1	1,749
p	<.001		<.001		NS		.001		
ES (*d*)	0.99		0.96		−0.07		−0.18		
Oppositional defiant disorder	21.1	0.8	21.6	0.8	5.9	0.4	6.3	0.4	28
Controls	13.6	0.1	12.3	0.1	6.3	<0.1	8.3	<0.1	1,894
p	<.001		<.001		NS		<.001		
ES (*d*)	1.14		1.26		−0.14		−0.54		
Conduct disorder	16.9	2.0	19.9	1.9	9.4	0.8	11.2	1.1	5
Controls	13.7	0.1	12.4	0.1	6.3	<0.1	8.3	<0.1	1,917
p	NS		<.001		<.001		.007		
ES (*d*)	0.63		0.90		0.70		0.51		
Any anxiety disorder	15.7	0.6	15.3	0.6	7.1	0.2	9.6	0.3	56
Controls	13.6	0.1	12.3	0.1	6.3	<0.1	8.2	<0.1	1,866
p	.001		<.001		.001		<.001		
ES (*d*)	0.30		0.42		0.24		0.31		
Any depressive disorder	15.2	0.8	14.1	0.8	6.8	0.3	10.1	0.4	32
Controls	13.7	0.1	12.4	0.1	6.3	<0.1	8.3	<0.1	1,890
p	NS		NS		NS		<.001		
ES (*d*)	0.23		0.23		0.16		0.45		
Bipolar disorder	15.9	1.2	16.5	1.1	7.9	0.5	10.6	0.6	14
Controls	13.7	0.1	12.4	0.1	6.3	<0.1	8.3	<0.1	1,908
p	NS		<.001		.001		<.001		
ES (*d*)	0.31		0.50		0.38		0.44		

(continued)

TABLE 6.2. *(continued)*

	ADHD Scores				SCT Scores				
	IN		HI		Daydreamy		Sluggish		
Diagnostic groups	Mean	*SE*	Mean	*SE*	Mean	*SE*	Mean	*SE*	*n*
Autism spectrum disorder	17.1	0.7	16.1	0.7	7.9	0.3	8.8	0.4	36
Controls	13.6	0.1	12.4	0.1	6.3	<0.1	8.3	<0.1	1,886
p	<.001		<.001		<.001		NS		
ES (*d*)	0.47		0.54		0.46		0.14		

Note. Listed in this table are each of the developmental and psychiatric diagnoses reported by parents in the U.S. normative sample in which the SCT total score served as the covariate for both ADHD scores, and the ADHD total score served as the covariate for both SCT scores. ADHD IN, ADHD Inattention symptom score; ADHD HI, ADHD Hyperactivity–Impulsivity symptom score; *SE*, standard error for the marginal (adjusted) mean; *F*, results for the *F*-test from the analysis of variance; *p*, probability value for each of the multivariate initial *F*-tests was $p \leq .001$ and follow-up univariate *F*-tests was $p \leq .05$; NS, not significant; ES (*d*), effect size calculated with Cohen's *d*, using the difference between the *adjusted* (marginal) means for each diagnostic group and the *unadjusted* standard deviations for each group. $N = 1{,}922$ for the normative sample.

zure, or autistic spectrum disorders (again, after controlling for ADHD symptoms) whereas the Sluggish dimension was not. In contrast, the Sluggish dimension of SCT was significantly *lower* in children with ADHD or ODD than in control cases, whereas no differences were evident from control cases for these two disorders on the SCT Daydreamy dimension. Recall that these analyses involved removal of any overlap of ADHD symptoms with these SCT factors. This is evidence of a double dissociation, in that findings for ADHD symptoms in these two disorders are the opposite of those for SCT symptom dimensions. These results are also consistent with some research showing that when the overlap with ADHD symptoms is removed, a negative relationship may exist between the SCT Sluggish dimension and ADHD, especially Hyperactivity–Impulsivity (see Chapter 1).

Patterns of Effect Sizes for SCT Symptoms within and across Disorders

Statistical significance is not the only or best means of conveying patterns of deficits within and across disorders for the ADHD and SCT symptom dimensions. That is because levels of statistical significance can be greatly affected by sample sizes in which small effects can be significant due to large samples, and vice versa. Hence it is better to examine the effect sizes for the various BSCTS-CA scores. It is possible to take the results from the analyses used to create Table 6.2 for each disorder and compute effect sizes (Cohen's *d*; Cohen, 1992) to create a common or standardized metric on which to compare the results within and across disorders. It also permits us to obtain some idea of which disorders are most likely to be associated with more severe levels of ADHD vs. SCT symptoms and how that association may differ across disorders. In this context an effect size is the difference in the adjusted mean scores (adjusted for the covariate) between each disorder and the control group, divided by the pooled raw standard deviations (for both the disordered and control groups). It is therefore the number of standard deviations that separate the mean scores for each disorder from the general population sample not having that disorder. Recall that the means used here are adjusted or estimated marginal means, as shown in Table 6.2, with scores for the other attention condition statistically removed (covaried). For instance, the SCT Total Symptom Score was removed from the means for the ADHD symptom dimensions, and vice versa.

This method of presenting results brings into sharper relief the magnitude of differences between the disordered and nondisordered groups in their ADHD and SCT symptoms, controlling for any overlap between these attention disorders. What do we see in these results? Effect sizes of 0.20+ are considered small, those of 0.50+ are considered moderate, and those of 0.80+ are considered large (Cohen, 1992).

Differences in children with and without physical disabilities were very modest and were not significant. The magnitude of the differences in symptoms of the two attention disorders for children with language delays was small and comparable for ADHD and SCT. Group differences for children with motor delays were larger and of a medium magnitude for ADHD Inattention (IN) and of small and comparable sizes for ADHD Hyperactive–Impulsive (HI) and both SCT dimensions.

What about the various LDs? In contrast to the preceding patterns, for children with diagnoses of reading disorders, both symptom dimensions of ADHD showed a far larger magnitude than was the case for both SCT dimensions, which were not significant. And symptoms of ADHD IN were of a medium magnitude and nearly twice that for ADHD HI symptoms. Thus, it is ADHD IN that is much more aligned with reading disorders, and to a lesser extent so are ADHD HI symptoms, than is the case for SCT symptoms. Similarly, for math disorders, ADHD IN once again showed the largest magnitude, having a medium effect size. But in contrast to reading disorders, differences in the ADHD HI symptoms were modest and not significant. Also, in contrast to reading disorders, symptoms of SCT were of a greater magnitude, though still of a small degree. Not surprisingly given their association with reading disorders, spelling disorders showed a comparable pattern to reading disorders with the greatest difference being in ADHD IN (medium magnitude), whereas the difference in ADHD HI symptoms were less than half this magnitude—and those for SCT were modest and not significant. A similar though not identical pattern was evident for writing disorders, where again ADHD IN showed the largest difference with a medium effect size, and ADHD HI was less than half that size, as was the SCT Daydreamy scale. SCT Sluggish symptoms were modest and not significant. This same pattern held true for children diagnosed with other academic disorders. So it is really ADHD IN symptoms that are most closely associated with the various learning disorders, having differences from controls that are of a moderate magnitude. SCT symptoms are not as substantial in these disorders and, where significant, are primarily limited to the SCT Daydreamy dimension and of a small magnitude.

In contrast, children diagnosed with general developmental delay or intellectual disability had more substantial differences in their symptoms, which were mostly of a medium size (except for ADHD HI, which was small in degree) and were comparable to ADHD IN and both SCT dimensions. Contrast this with the pattern for tic disorders, for which ADHD HI symptoms were of the greatest and medium magnitude, with ADHD IN and the two SCT dimensions being of a much smaller magnitude and not significant. For children diagnosed with seizure disorders, only SCT Daydreamy symptoms were significant and at a medium effect size.

A pattern of larger effect sizes was evident for the more classic or traditional psychiatric disorders of childhood, than was evident for the earlier developmental, learning, and neurological disorders. For children diagnosed with ADHD, the magnitude of both ADHD symptom dimensions was of a large size and more than 10 times greater than that seen for SCT, where SCT Daydreamy was not significant and SCT Sluggish symptoms were of a negative but modest magnitude. These findings clearly validate both the distinction between ADHD and SCT as attention disorders and also the SCT scores from BSCTS-CA scales. For ODD, even larger effect sizes were evident on the two ADHD symptom dimensions, indeed being the greatest in magnitude across all disorders in Table 6.2. This finding is not unexpected, given that ODD is associated with an increased severity of ADHD symptoms in children diagnosed with ADHD (Angold et al., 1999; Brown, 2009). In contrast, SCT Daydreamy is not associated with ODD once its overlap with ADHD is removed. And notice that the magnitude of the differences for the SCT Slow symptoms is not only of a medium degree but is in a *negative* direction. This means that, controlling for the overlap with ADHD symptoms, SCT Sluggish symptoms are less likely to occur in children with ODD than even in typically developing (control) children. As noted in Chapter 1, this double dissociation or negative relationship of SCT to ODD symptoms has been observed previously once any overlap of SCT with ADHD is removed. This is clear evidence not only that SCT is distinct from both ADHD and ODD, but that the BSCTS-CA scales assessing SCT are capable of detecting this dissociation. The pattern for conduct disorder was different from that evident in ODD. Here, all symptom dimensions of ADHD and SCT had differences of medium to large effect sizes and of a positive direction or valence.

Group differences for all SCT scores from the BSCTS-CA for the internalizing and mood disorders were of a far lower magnitude than for ADHD, ODD, and conduct disorder, being of small magnitude. For anxiety disorders, the differences were significant but of a small degree and relatively comparable for both ADHD and SCT symptoms scores. Not so for depression, for which the effect sizes for both ADHD dimensions and SCT Daydreamy, while small, were not significant. Only the SCT Sluggish dimension was significant and of a small-to-medium magnitude. Again, this result is similar to that discussed in Chapter 1, where prior research suggests that it is SCT symptoms that are linked to depression, not ADHD symptoms. The present findings clarify this association, further implying that it is mainly the SCT Sluggish symptom set that drives this relationship. For bipolar disorder, the link to elevated ADHD symptoms was for the HI dimension only and of a medium effect size. Both SCT dimensions were associated with bipolar disorder and of a small-to-medium effect size. In contrast, group differences for children with an autistic spectrum disorder (ASD) were evident on both ADHD dimensions and of a medium effect size, which was also the case for the SCT Daydreamy symptoms, whereas SCT Sluggish symptoms were not significantly associated with ASD.

The Likelihood of Children with Clinically Deviant Scores on SCT Scales

Having a Developmental, Learning, or Psychiatric Diagnosis

Probably a more clinically meaningful way to demonstrate the validity of the BSCTS-CA ratings is to select children who score significantly above normal, or in the clinically deviant range of the population, in their SCT ratings. One can then determine the extent to which these children experienced various types of developmental, learning, and psychiatric diagnoses, as reported by parents in the national survey. If the ratings on the BSCTS-CA are reasonably valid, then children so identified should have a significantly greater likelihood of having SCT, given that comorbidity among disorders is commonplace (Angold et al., 1999). For these purposes, the score at the 93rd percentile for the SCT Total Score was used to make this determination. The 93rd percentile is used here because it is commonly used in research and with other rating scales of child behavior to determine a clinically significant score. Chi-square analyses were then employed to determine the percentage of children having a clinically elevated SCT score who had any of the noted diagnoses. This type of analysis is the inverse of the information presented in the preceding sections, yet is more consistent with how a clinician is likely to use the BSCTS-CA. The clinician will have obtained the ratings on this scale initially and will then wish to know the extent to which significantly high scores on it place the child at risk—in this case, at risk for certain diagnoses. The results are shown in Table 6.3.

TABLE 6.3. Percentages of Cases Having Clinically Elevated (High) SCT Total Score and Clinically Elevated ADHD Total Score and Respective Control Groups (Low SCT, Low ADHD) Having Various Professionally Diagnosed Disorders as Reported by Parents

	Groups (percentages)					
Prior diagnosis	Low SCT	High SCT	χ^2	Low ADHD	High ADHD	χ^2
Language delay	4.2	15.5	35.61[a]	4.0	17.6	51.36[a]
Delayed motor skills–coordination	2.5	12.7	42.72[a]	2.2	16.9	89.76[a]
Reading disorder	3.4	11.3	21.02[a]	3.0	16.9	66.97[a]
Math disorder	1.9	7.0	15.48[a]	1.6	10.6	46.93[a]
Spelling disorder	1.9	7.7	19.59[a]	1.9	8.5	25.03[a]
Writing disorder	1.6	9.9	40.72[a]	1.5	11.3	57.17[a]
Other learning disorders	1.4	5.6	13.94[a]	1.1	9.2	50.27[a]
General delay–intellectual disability	0.6	8.5	72.33[a]	0.4	9.9	102.90
Tic disorders/Tourette syndrome	0.5	1.4	1.88	0.4	2.1	6.39
Deaf/hard of hearing	0.3	2.1	10.46[a]	0.3	1.4	3.64
Blind/very visually impaired	0.3	4.2	32.04[a]	0.3	4.9	45.80[a]
ADD/ADHD	7.6	26.8	59.04[a]	5.4	53.5	371.03[a]
ODD	1.5	1.4	<0.01	0.6	12.0	118.09[a]
Conduct disorder	0.1	2.8	38.63[a]	0.1	2.8	38.63[a]
Any anxiety disorder	2.3	10.6	31.72[a]	1.9	15.5	85.77[a]
Any depressive disorder	1.2	7.0	27.08[a]	1.3	6.3	20.45[a]
Bipolar disorder	0.4	4.2	25.93[a]	0.4	4.9	37.42[a]
Autism or autistic spectrum disorder	1.1	11.3	73.63[a]	1.0	12.7	97.36[a]
None of the above disorders	80.1	45.8	88.70[a]	81.3	29.6	202.28

Note. Low SCT, SCT Total Score < 93rd percentile based on entire normative sample (N = 1,780); High SCT, SCT Total Score ≥ 93rd percentile (N = 142); Low ADHD, ADHD Total Score < 93rd percentile (N = 1,780); High ADHD, ADHD Total Score ≥ 93rd percentile (N = 142); χ^2 = results of the chi-square test.

[a] $p \leq .001$.

As Table 6.3 indicates, children with High SCT Total Scores were at a significantly greater risk for having most of the disorders in the table, although the percentages for each disorder were fairly low in an absolute sense. Yet those risks were still higher than the population risk, as identified in the control or Low SCT group. The most frequent disorder was, not surprisingly, ADHD/ADD followed by language delays, motor coordination disorders, reading disorders, ASD, and anxiety disorders. Noteworthy is the finding that High and Low SCT groups did not differ significantly in their risk for ODD—a finding consistent with research presented in Chapter 1. About 54% of the High SCT group had one or more of the disorders shown in the table, compared to 20% of the Low SCT group.

When comparing cases that scored high on ADHD symptoms in the national survey to those scoring below the 93rd percentile, a similar pattern for risk emerges as it did with SCT. This is not unexpected, given that SCT and ADHD have some relationship to each other and that nearly half of children having one condition (ADHD) have the other (SCT), and vice versa (Barkley, 2013). There were a few exceptions. High ADHD scorers, of course, not only had a far greater risk for an ADHD/ADD diagnosis than did those with Low ADHD Total Scores but also far higher than those having High SCT Total Scores. The High ADHD group also had a much greater risk for ODD, which, as noted, was not an elevated risk at all associated with High SCT scorers. In general, High ADHD scorers had a 70% chance of having at least one of the disorders in Table 6.3, again compared to just 20% for the Low ADHD group and well above that risk seen in the High SCT group (54%).

Conclusions

This chapter has provided a large body of evidence in support of the validity of the BSCTS-CA for evaluating SCT in the daily life activities of children. Whether it is for construct, convergent, divergent, or criterion validity, the evidence is sufficient to validate this rating scale and its subscale scores. The most clinically and scientifically informative evidence for the utility of the BSCTS-CA comes from the abundant evidence that it can readily distinguish various patterns of symptoms in daily life across various neurodevelopmental, learning, and psychiatric disorders of childhood. It does so beyond the far easier hurdle of differentiating between various disordered groups and a control group not having that disorder. Such evidence shows the BSCTS-CA has considerable utility both in clinical practice, where individuals with such disorders must be evaluated, but also in research into the nature and correlates of these two attention disorders. The results provided here also lend confidence to the effort to conduct more rigorous investigations into the nature of SCT.

CHAPTER 7

Relationships of BSCTS-CA Scores to Impairments

As has been noted previously (Barkley, 2011c), symptoms and impairments are not identical and do not have a perfect or direct relationship with each other. Symptoms can be viewed as the cognitions and behaviors associated with and arising from a particular disorder, such as ADHD or SCT. Impairments are the consequences of displaying those behaviors to such an extent that they lead to functional ineffectiveness in particular domains of major life activities. The items on the BSCTS-CA can be largely, if not entirely, conceptualized as symptoms of SCT. They are clearly not impairments, in and of themselves, by this definition. This chapter examines the relationship of such symptoms to the degree of functional ineffectiveness and the adverse consequences that ensue as a result of variation in the severity of those attention disorders and their symptoms—in short, it examines degree of impairment in relation to severity of SCT symptoms. I begin with an obvious set of measures of impairment: the extent to which the children in the national survey were rated as being functionally ineffective by their parents, both in 15 domains of life activities and more globally. Is the type of impairment in any way related to the severity of SCT symptoms, as reflected across the BSCTS-CA subscales?

In some of the analyses in the previous chapter, the severity of ADHD was statistically removed (covaried) when examining the effects of SCT, or vice versa (or ADHD). This makes sense when trying to examine the construct, the convergent and divergent validity of the two disorders of interest, and the SCT scales of the BSCTS-CA with their underlying dimensions. I was trying to show the distinctiveness of each disorder from the other. However, here I am examining the concurrent or ecological validity of the BSCTS-CA scores and their utility in assessing a child's risk for other problems or correlates of the disorders. This is just what a clinician will do when examining the results for a particular patient. In short, what do high scores on these SCT scales mean for the child or teen? In doing so, the clinician will certainly not statistically covary the results of one set of attention disorder scores, such as for ADHD, out of those scores for the other attention disorder, such as SCT. Therefore, no ANOVAs using ADHD scores as covariates are reported here, so that these results can be directly applied to interpreting high scores on the BSCTS-CA subscales, as will be done in routine clinical practice.

Specific and Global Ratings of Impairment

Relationship of SCT Ratings to Impairment Ratings

Impairment was assessed more directly in the original sample by having parents complete a rating scale assessing degree of psychosocial impairment in 15 domains of major life activities on the Barkley Functional Impairment Scale—Children and Adolescents (BFIS-CA; Barkley, 2012b). On this scale, each domain is rated on a 0 (not at all) to 9 (severely impaired) Likert scaling. Parents also indicated if any domain was not applicable for their child. Such responses were treated as missing data in the correlation analyses. These ratings of impairment were then correlated with the four BSCTS-CA scores as another indicator of criterion validity. The results for these Pearson product–moment correlations are shown in Table 7.1. All correlations were of a moderate magnitude and significant (all $ps < .001$), which is not surprising given the large sample size. The pattern of scores is informative and provides yet more evidence of validity of the BSCTS-CA SCT scores. Results for the SCT scores were uniform across the various domains of impairment. The SCT scores share about 10–30% of the variance with those impairment ratings.

Extent of Impairment in Children with High SCT Ratings

Probably a more clinically meaningful way to demonstrate the validity of the BSCTS-CA ratings is to select children who score significantly above normal, or in the clinically deviant range of the population, in their SCT ratings. We can then determine the extent to which these children experienced various forms of impairment. If the ratings are reasonably valid, then children so identified should have significantly more impairment and more types of impairment than do the children placing below that threshold. For these purposes, the same procedure was followed as in the prior chapter: The score at the 93rd percentile for the SCT Total Score was used to determine if a child was clinically deviant in either of these sets of symptoms.

In the survey, if parents had endorsed at least one or more items as occurring "often" or "very often" on the ratings of SCT, they were asked to indicate whether or not those symptoms interfered with their child's functioning in any of four different domains of life activities: these being Home, Social relations, School, and Community activities. Chi-square analyses were used initially to compare children with clinically elevated SCT Total Scores.

The results showed that 39% of the parents who had endorsed at least one symptom of SCT for their child (answer of "often" or "very often") but who were not clinically deviant in their total SCT rating (Low SCT, $N = 204$) described their

TABLE 7.1. Correlations of BSCTS-CA SCT Scores with Ratings on 15 Domains of Impairment from the BFIS-CA

	SCT scores			
BFIS-CA domains	DD	SL	Total	SC
With Mother	.40	.38	.41	.34
With Father	.40	.40	.43	.36
School Performance	.52	.47	.53	.45
With Siblings	.45	.42	.46	.40
Other Children	.48	.43	.49	.43
Community Activities	.47	.46	.49	.43
Visiting Others	.51	.48	.52	.47
Playing at School	.49	.45	.50	.44
Managing Money	.41	.38	.42	.35
Self-Care	.48	.48	.51	.47
Doing Chores	.49	.46	.51	.42
School Homework	.50	.47	.52	.44
Following Rules	.50	.48	.52	.47
Other Adults	.49	.48	.52	.47
Playing Sports	.47	.47	.50	.52

Note. Analyses are Pearson product–moment correlations. All correlations are significant at $p < .001$. Sample sizes for correlations range from 1,607 to 1,824. DD, SCT Daydreamy Score; SL, SCT Sluggish Score; Total, SCT Total Score; SC, Symptom Count Score.

child's symptoms as interfering with Home functioning. The figure for the High SCT symptom group ($N = 102$) was nearly twice that, at 71% ($\chi^2 = 27.05$, $p < .001$). Similar results were seen in comparing the Low and High SCT symptom groups in Social relations (37 vs. 68%, respectively; $\chi^2 = 25.42$, $p < .001$), School functioning (58 vs. 80%, respectively; $\chi^2 = 14.59$, $p < .001$), and Community activities (29 vs. 46%, respectively; $\chi^2 = 8.29$, $p = .004$).

Remember that many children having Low SCT ratings are not in these comparisons because their parents did not endorse at least one symptom as occurring often or very often. And so those parents were not asked to rate their child's functional interference in these four domains. Therefore, this Low SCT group should be considered symptomatic to some extent nonetheless. The fact that parents who did not endorse at least one symptom as occurring often or very often were not asked to rate their child's functional interference accounts for the seemingly higher-than-expected percentage of children in the Low SCT group that experienced some functional ineffectiveness in a specific domain. If all children who were in the Low SCT group and not at all symptomatic were added to these analyses, results would show that just 8% of the Low SCT group ($N = 1{,}780$) were rated as symptomatic *and* functionally impaired in at least one domain, compared to 63% of those in the High SCT group (χ^2 = 374.26, $p < .001$). Over all, having clinically elevated ratings of SCT on the BSCTS-CA places a child at significantly greater risk of having impaired functioning across all four domains of major life activities. On average, children with elevated SCT scores who were symptomatic were experiencing functional interference in at least 2.6 (SD = 1.4) of the four domains, compared to 1.6 domains in the Low SCT but symptomatic group (SD = 1.4; F = 35.29; df = 1,304; $p < .001$).

Specific Domains of Impairment for Children with Elevated SCT Symptoms

As noted previously, parents also completed a rating scale of impairment concerning 15 domains of daily life activities, the BFIS-CA. For each domain, parents rated the child on a 0–9 Likert scale as to the child's degree of functional ineffectiveness in that domain. One can therefore compare all children in the national sample rated as Low or High in SCT symptoms on these ratings for each of the domains of impairment. The results for these SCT groups are shown in Table 7.2. The groups

TABLE 7.2. Comparison of Children Who Did (High) or Did Not (Low) Place in the Clinically Elevated Range on the SCT Total Score on the 15 Domains from the BFIS-CA

	Low SCT (N = 1,097)		High SCT (N = 66)			
BFIS-CA Domain	Mean	*SD*	Mean	*SD*	*F*	*p*
With Mother	0.8	1.7	3.6	2.7	157.44	<.001
With Father	0.8	1.8	3.8	2.6	157.91	<.001
School Performance	0.9	1.9	4.6	2.7	219.44	<.001
With Siblings	1.0	1.8	3.9	2.8	143.33	<.001
Other Children	0.7	1.5	3.7	2.8	226.95	<.001
Community Activities	0.6	1.4	3.5	2.6	244.06	<.001
Visiting Others	0.5	1.3	3.3	2.6	244.29	<.001
Playing at School	0.6	1.5	3.5	2.7	198.15	<.001
Managing Money	0.8	1.6	3.5	2.7	158.73	<.001
Self-Care	0.6	1.4	3.5	3.0	231.39	<.001
Doing Chores	1.2	1.8	4.4	2.9	176.66	<.001
School Homework	1.1	1.9	4.5	2.9	175.72	<.001
Following Rules	0.8	1.7	4.2	2.9	212.13	<.001
Other Adults	0.5	1.3	3.4	2.6	248.44	<.001
Playing Sports	0.7	1.6	3.8	2.8	210.39	<.001

Note. F, results for the univariate F-test if multivariate F-test was significant ($p < .001$); p, probability value for the univariate F-test if $\leq .01$.

were initially compared using a multivariate analysis of variance (MANOVA), given that there is some correlation expected among the impairment ratings. The multivariate *F*-test was significant ($F = 22.75$; $df = 15{,}1147$; $p < .001$). Univariate ANOVAs were then used to compare groups on each of the 15 domains. The results indicated that children scoring high in their SCT symptoms were significantly and substantially more impaired, as rated by their parents in all of the 15 domains, than were children who were low in their SCT ratings. This rating scale also provides for three summary scores, reflecting the mean rating across those domains falling in the Home–School (work) domains, the mean rating across the Community–Leisure domains, and the number of the 15 domains rated in the impaired range (≥ 93rd percentile). Those results were also significant. Again, children rated as high in SCT symptoms ($N = 136$) had significantly greater mean ratings of impairment than those low in SCT symptoms ($N = 1{,}697$) in both the Home–School domains (mean = 4.0 vs. 1.1, *SD*s = 2.3 vs. 1.6, $F = 352.74$, $p < .001$) and the Community–Leisure domains (mean = 3.6 vs. 0.7, *SD*s = 2.4 vs. 1.4, $F = 428.09$, $p < .001$). Those in the High SCT group were rated as being impaired in at least an average of 4.4 domains compared to 0.7 for the Low SCT group (*SD*s = 4.4 vs. 2.0, $F = 293.44$, $p < .001$).

The relationship of the SCT Symptom Count score to the risk for impairment in these same domains is shown in Figure 7.1. Here I have combined the SCT Daydreamy and SCT Sluggish symptom counts into a single symptom count score, as reflected in the scoring of the BSCTS-CA where only a total symptom count is com-

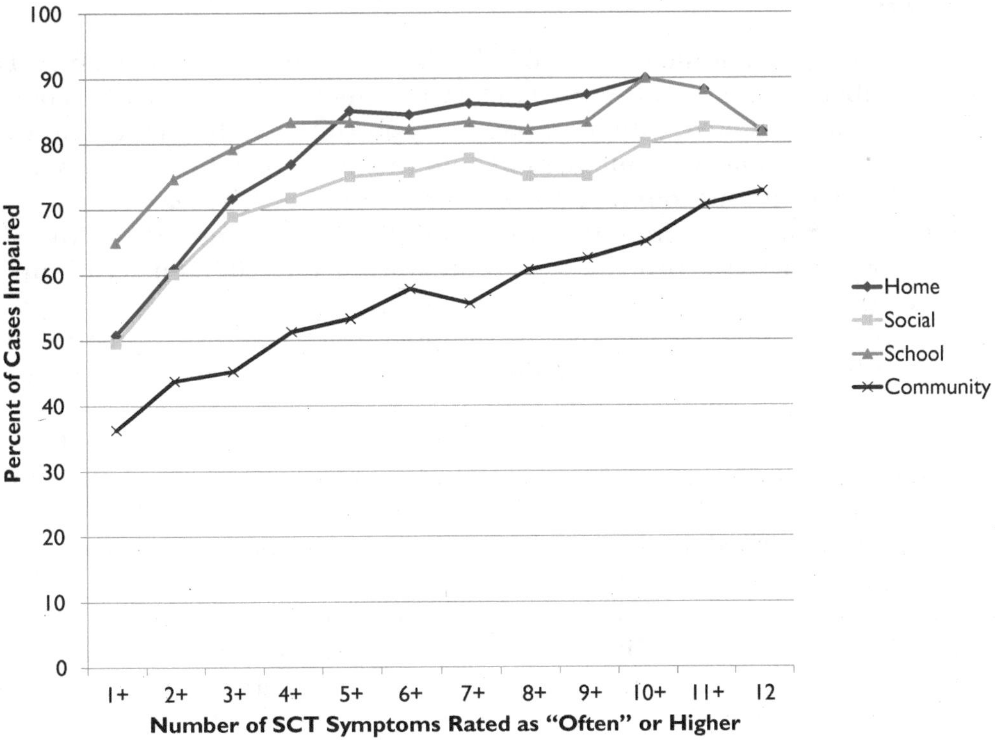

FIGURE 7.1. Percentage of cases reported to be impaired in each of four domains (Home, Social, School, and Community) for each Symptom Count Score of SCT symptoms.

puted across all 12 symptoms. The risk of impairment is significantly increased with each rise in SCT Symptom Counts, especially in the Home setting, such that by four or more symptoms, 80% or more of cases at this or higher symptom counts are said to be impaired in School, and by five or more symptoms, 80% are impaired in the Home setting. In contrast, it takes 10 or more symptoms to hit this level of risk (80%) in the Social domain and 11 or more to do so in the Community domain.

All of these findings indicate that the more elevated the scores for SCT ratings on the BSCTS-CA, the greater is the risk for impairment in various domains of major life activities. High BSCTS-CA scores are also associated with impairment in many more such domains than is the case for children not placing in the clinically deviant range on these scores. This is even more evidence for the validity of the BSCTS-CA scores.

Specific Areas of Psychosocial Impairment

Parents in the original sample were also asked questions about specific areas of important psychosocial adjustment as another indicator of potential impairment in their children. The relationship of BSCTS-CA scores to each of these areas of psychosocial impairment examined in this section for further evidence of validity of the scale scores.

Friendships

Parents were asked about the number of friends their children had currently. The range of numbers of friends was from 0 to 99 with a mean = 7.7 ($SD = 8.4$). The distribution was highly skewed, with most parents reporting that their child had from 3 to 10 friends, with a median number of 5 and the mode of 5. Correlations of the number of friends with the four SCT scores were –.08 for the SCT Daydreamy score, –.08 for the SCT Sluggish score, –.08 for the SCT Total Score, and –.07 for the SCT Symptom Count score. All correlations were significant at $p < .001$, but clearly are of a modest degree.

Given the substantial skew of this distribution, which can distort a correlation coefficient, a better way of portraying the relationship of the BSCTS-CA scores to this domain of impairment is to subdivide the sample into those having 1 or no friends to those with 2 or more. Having 1 or fewer friends represents the bottom 5.7% of the population sample. It could be taken as an index of impairment in friendships with other children and certainly as a marker of unpopularity. A total of 108 children comprised this Unpopular group and were compared to the remainder of the sample on the eight BSCTS-CA subscales. The results are shown in Table 7.3. Clearly, higher BSCTS-CA scores are associated with being in the Unpopular group, with effect sizes placing in the medium range. That makes sense, given the importance of SCT behaviors for sustaining friendships with others. An alternative means of examining this relationship of BSCTS-CA scores to friendships is by evaluating the percentage of children placing in the clinically deficient range on the SCT Total Score of the BSCTS-CA who also placed in the Unpopular group just discussed. Results indicated that children in the clinical range on the SCT Total

TABLE 7.3. Comparison of Unpopular Children (Who Had One or Fewer Friends) with Popular Children (Two or More Friends) on the SCT Subscale Scores of the BSCTS-CA

	Popular (N = 1,797)		Unpopular (N = 108)				
	Mean	*SD*	Mean	*SD*	*F*	*p*	ES (*d*)
SCT Daydreamy Score	6.2	2.2	8.1	3.7	68.35	<.001	0.62
SCT Sluggish Score	8.2	2.7	10.3	4.5	58.26	<.001	0.54
SCT Total Score	14.4	4.6	18.4	7.6	71.95	<.001	0.64
SCT Symptom Count Score	0.4	1.4	1.5	2.8	56.51	<.001	0.50

Note. F, results for the univariate *F*-test; *p*, probability value for the univariate *F*-test if ≤.05; ES (*d*), effect size for mean differences (treated vs. untreated) computed as Cohen's *d*.

Score (N = 140) were approximately 4 times more likely to place in the Unpopular group than were children in the Low SCT group (N = 1,765) (18.4 vs. 4.6%, respectively; $\chi^2 = 47.04$, $p < .001$).

Community Activities

Parents reported the number of clubs, sports, church groups, and organizations their children had belonged to in the previous year. The mean number was 2.2 (*SD* = 2.3) (median = 2, mode = 2). A total of 89% of children belonged to four or fewer such community organizations. The correlations between the BSCTS-CA SCT subscale scores and the number of community organizations or clubs to which the child belonged ranged from –.08 (SCT Daydreamy) to –.12 (SCT Total Score), with all being significant at $p < .001$. These are very modest correlations, but they do show some relationship of SCT scores to participation in Community activities.

Parents were also asked to report the number of formal organized sports in which their child participated in the past year, apart from the physical education classes at school. The mean was 1.2 (*SD* = 1.4) (median = 1, mode = 0). The correlations between the BSCTS-CA scores and the sports participation ranged from –.12 to –.14 for the four SCT scores, all being significant (all *p*s < .001), albeit of a modest magnitude. As with clubs and other organized community activities, there is a small but significant negative relationship between SCT, as rated by parents, and sports participation.

School Grades

Parents in the original sample were asked to indicate their child's letter grades (or percentages corresponding to those grades), as reported on their previous report card, using the following response categories: A (90–100%), B (80–89%), C (70–79%), D (60–69%), and E or F (50–59% or failing). A total of 1,861 parents provided information to this question as follows: A = 54%, B = 32%, C = 11%, D = 2%, and F = 1%. The correlations (Pearson *r*s) between the SCT scores on the BSCTS-CA and this measure were SCT Daydreamy = .28, SCT Sluggish = .30, SCT Total

Score = .31, and SCT Symptom Count = .26 (all *p*s < .001). Thus, SCT scores share up to approximately 9% of the variance with parental reports of their child's GPA.

Another way of illustrating this relationship is to compare children who placed in the C or lower range of grades (14% of sample) against those who had an A or B average on their BSCTS-CA. This comparison is shown in Table 7.4. The univariate ANOVAs comparing the groups on the four BSCTS-CA scores were all significant as well at the $p < .001$ level. Obviously, children with letter grades of C or lower have significantly higher BSCTS-CA subscale scores than those with grades of A or B. The effect sizes were of a medium magnitude for all SCT scores.

Another way of examining this relationship that is more clinically meaningful is to ask what percentage of cases that placed in the clinically deviant range on SCT Total Scores had a grade of C or lower. For SCT, those scoring High ($N = 130$) were 3.5 times more likely to have a grade of C or lower than were those Low in SCT ($N = 1{,}731$) (41.5 vs. 11.6%, respectively; $\chi^2 = 92.24$, $p < .001$). As noted here, SCT is not a benign condition with regard to school functioning.

School Adjustment

Information was also available from parents on whether or not their child's teachers had told the parents during the past year that their child was having significant problems with his/her behavior or school performance. A comparison of the 501 children receiving such a report to the 1,409 children who did not showed that the former were having significantly more problems with SCT symptoms in daily school life. The results of these comparisons are shown in Table 7.5 for all four BSCTS-CA scores. Univariate ANOVAs were used to compare the groups on the four BSCTS-CA scores, with all comparisons being significant (all *p*s < .001). It is obvious from the results that SCT scores were in the medium range.

Again, one can ask the more clinically meaningful question: What percentage of cases that placed in the clinically deviant range on SCT Total Scores had received recent teacher complaints about their behavior or schoolwork. For SCT, those scoring High ($N = 140$) were 2.5 times more likely to have had a teacher complaint about these matters recently than were those Low in SCT ($N = 1{,}770$) (60.7 vs. 23.5%,

TABLE 7.4. Comparison of Children Having Letter Grades of A or B with Children Having a Grade of C or Lower on the SCT Subscale Scores of the BSCTS-CA

	Grade = A or B ($N = 1{,}607$)		Grade = ≤ C ($N = 254$)				
	Mean	*SD*	Mean	*SD*	*F*	*p*	ES (*d*)
SCT Daydreamy Score	6.0	1.9	7.8	3.5	135.68	<.001	0.64
SCT Sluggish Score	7.9	2.3	10.4	4.7	172.65	<.001	0.67
SCT Total Score	14.0	3.9	18.2	7.9	179.68	<.001	0.64
SCT Symptom Count Score	0.3	1.1	1.4	2.9	129.90	<.001	0.50

Note. F, results for the univariate *F*-test; *p* = probability value for the univariate *F*-test if ≤.05; ES (*d*), effect size for mean differences (treated vs. untreated) computed as Cohen's *d*.

TABLE 7.5. Comparison of Children Whose Teachers Did Not Report a Problem with Behavior or Schoolwork to Those Whose Teachers Did So on the SCT Subscale Scores of the BSCTS-CA

	No Problems (N = 1,409)		Problems in School (N = 501)				
	Mean	*SD*	Mean	*SD*	*F*	*p*	ES (*d*)
SCT Daydreamy Score	5.8	1.6	7.6	3.3	248.22	<.001	0.69
SCT Sluggish Score	7.8	2.0	9.7	4.2	185.62	<.001	0.58
SCT Total Score	13.6	3.2	17.3	7.1	246.26	<.001	0.67
SCT Symptom Count Score	0.2	0.8	1.1	2.6	152.43	<.001	0.47

Note. F, results for the univariate *F*-test; *p*, probability value for the univariate *F*-test if ≤.05; ES (*d*), effect size for mean differences (treated vs. untreated) computed as Cohen's *d*.

respectively; $\chi^2 = 92.84$, $p < .001$). This evidence concerning school adjustment is consistent with related evidence presented above and in Chapter 1. Again, SCT has an impairing effect in the School domain. Once more, these findings provide considerable evidence for the validity of the BSCTS-CA scores.

Parents were also asked if their children had ever been retained in grade. There were 102 children who had been so retained, and they were compared to the remainder (N = 1,812) on the BSCTS-CA subscale scores. Again, univariate ANOVAs were computed to compare these two groups on all four BSCTS-CA scores. The results appear in Table 7.6. All comparisons were significant at $p < .001$. Here we can see that children who had been retained had significantly more SCT symptoms than did those who had never been retained a grade in school.

Even more clinically informative was the comparison of the groups scoring High in SCT symptoms to those scoring low in their risk for grade retention. Those scoring high (N = 140) were about 3 times more likely to have been retained in a grade than were those Low in SCT (N = 1,774) (15.7 vs. 4.5%, respectively; χ^2 = 32.29, $p < .001$). Hence, clinically elevated levels of SCT appear to convey risk for grade retention in school. Medium effect sizes can be noted in Table 7.6.

TABLE 7.6. Comparison of Children Who Had Been Retained in Grade to Those Who Had Not on the SCT Subscale Scores of the BSCTS-CA

	Not retained (N = 1,812)		Retained in grade (N = 501)				
	Mean	*SD*	Mean	*SD*	*F*	*p*	ES (*d*)
SCT Daydreamy Score	6.2	2.1	8.0	4.1	61.21	<.001	0.55
SCT Sluggish Score	8.2	2.7	10.0	5.2	40.47	<.001	0.43
SCT Total Score	14.4	4.5	18.1	8.9	56.39	<.001	0.52
SCT Symptom Count Score	0.4	1.4	1.5	3.3	56.60	<.001	0.43

Note. F, results for the univariate *F*-test; *p*, probability value for the univariate *F*-test if ≤.05; ES (*d*), effect size for mean differences (treated vs. untreated) computed as Cohen's *d*.

As another index of school adjustment, parents reported if their child had ever been suspended or expelled from school ($N = 129$) or not ($N = 1{,}783$). Once again, univariate ANOVAs comparing these two groups on all four BSCTS-CA scores were all significant as well ($p < .001$). The results appear in Table 7.7. Obviously, these results make it clear that children experiencing suspension or expulsion have higher SCT scores on all BSCTS-CA indices than do those who never experienced this adverse outcome in their educational careers. Effect sizes were medium for SCT.

The comparison of the groups scoring high in SCT symptoms to those scoring low in their risk for school suspension and expulsion found that those scoring high ($N = 139$) were about 2.5 times more likely to have been suspended or expelled than were those Low in SCT ($N = 1{,}773$) (16.5 vs. 6.0%, respectively; $\chi^2 = 22.88$, $p < .001$).

All of this evidence indicates that symptoms of SCT, as rated on the BSCTS-CA, are significantly related to various indices of school maladjustment (behavior or performance problems, grade retention, and suspensions/expulsions). Here again we find substantial evidence for the validity of the BSCTS-CA scores and for the impact of this attention disorder on school adjustment.

Accidental Injuries and Poisonings

Children with psychiatric disorders are known to be at increased risk for accidental injuries (Rowe, Maughan, & Goodman, 2004). After controlling for comorbidity with other disorders and some psychosocial risk factors, research shows that ODD may be more associated specifically with burns and poisonings, whereas ADHD is linked to risk for fractures (Rowe et al., 2004). Depression and anxiety may also be linked to certain injury types as well. Children with ADHD have been shown to be at a significantly increased risk (without controlling for comorbidity) for having accidental injuries of all types including poisonings (Barkley, 2015c; Hinshaw, 2002). Given that nearly all of the psychiatric disorders were found (in Chapter 7) to be linked to both attention disorders, it is likely that BSCTS-CA scores would be associated with accidental injuries or poisonings.

We asked parents to report on how many times their child had been taken to a doctor or hospital for treatment of an accidental injury or poisoning. The majority of children ($N = 1{,}309$; 69%) had never had such an event, whereas 18% had just one such event. About 5% had experienced three or more such events. This latter

TABLE 7.7. Comparison of Children Who Had Been Suspended or Expelled from School to Those Who Had Not on the SCT Subscale Scores of the BSCTS-CA

	Not suspended ($N = 1{,}783$)		Suspended/expelled ($N = 129$)				
	Mean	*SD*	Mean	*SD*	*F*	*p*	ES (*d*)
SCT Daydreamy Score	6.2	2.1	7.8	3.7	58.44	<.001	0.53
SCT Sluggish Score	8.1	2.6	10.2	4.8	62.35	<.001	0.54
SCT Total Score	14.3	4.5	18.0	8.1	69.61	<.001	0.56
SCT Symptom Count Score	0.4	1.4	1.4	3.0	58.51	<.001	0.43

Note. F, results for the univariate *F*-test; *p*, probability value for the univariate *F*-test if ≤.05; ES (*d*), effect size for mean differences (treated vs. untreated) computed as Cohen's *d*.

group was therefore considered to be injury prone. They were compared on the BSCTS-CA subscales to those having two or fewer such injuries/poisonings. The results are shown in Table 7.8, with all the comparisons. Again, univariate ANOVAs were computed to compare these two groups on all four BSCTS-CA scores, all of which were significant ($p < .001$). Children considered as accident prone by the preceding criterion had significantly more symptoms of SCT than did those not considered to be so prone. Effect sizes were of a small to medium magnitude.

As has been done for all measures of impairment in this chapter, I compared those scoring high in SCT symptoms ($N = 140$) with those low in SCT ($N = 1{,}765$) (10.7 vs. 4.4%, respectively; $\chi^2 = 11.07$, $p < .001$) and found that those who were high in SCT symptoms were about two times more likely to be considered accident prone. Thus, SCT conveys a twofold risk of being accident prone. Here again is evidence of the validity of the BSCTS-CA scores.

Relationship to Treatments

Psychiatric Medications

One obvious consequence or outcome that may be associated with having attention deficits from either ADHD or SCT may be the extent to which the child has been given psychiatric medications. There is every reason to suspect just such a relationship, given the findings in the previous chapter: ADHD and SCT symptoms are found in conjunction with many psychiatric and developmental disorders, and psychiatric medications are often used to treat such disorders, especially ADHD. Parents in the sample were asked if their child had ever been treated with a psychiatric medication for management of a psychiatric or psychological disorder. Children who had been so treated were compared to those not so treated on all four of the BSCTS-CA rating scores.

The univariate ANOVAs were computed for each of the scores. The results are shown in Table 7.9, where it is evident that children receiving medication for psychiatric disorders were more likely to manifest higher scores for the SCT scales and symptom count than those who did not receive that therapy (all ANOVAs were significant at $p < .001$). The effect sizes are substantial and are medium to large for SCT scores.

TABLE 7.8. Comparison of Children Who Were Accident Prone (Two or More Injuries) to Those Who Were Not on the SCT Subscale Scores of the BSCTS-CA

	Not prone (N = 1,812)		Accident prone (N = 93)				
	Mean	*SD*	Mean	*SD*	*F*	*p*	ES (*d*)
SCT Daydreamy Score	6.2	2.2	7.4	3.7	20.75	<.001	0.39
SCT Sluggish Score	8.2	2.7	9.7	4.9	22.88	<.001	0.38
SCT Total Score	14.5	4.6	17.1	8.2	25.11	<.001	0.39
SCT Symptom Count Score	0.4	1.5	1.2	2.9	23.38	<.001	0.35

Note. F, results for the univariate *F*-test; *p*, probability value for the univariate *F*-test if ≤.05; ES (*d*), effect size for mean differences (treated vs. untreated) computed as Cohen's *d*.

TABLE 7.9. Comparison of Children Who Had and Had Not Received Psychiatric Medication on the BSCTS-CA ADHD and SCT Subscale Scores

	No medication (N = 1,766)		Medication (N = 156)				
	Mean	*SD*	Mean	*SD*	*F*	*p*	ES (*d*)
SCT Daydreamy Score	6.1	2.0	8.4	3.8	154.86	<.001	0.76
SCT Sluggish Score	8.1	2.6	10.6	4.8	108.80	<.001	0.65
SCT Total Score	14.2	4.3	19.0	8.0	147.75	<.001	0.75
SCT Symptom Count Score	0.3	1.3	1.8	3.1	137.54	<.001	0.63

Note. F, results for the univariate *F*-test; *p*, probability value for the univariate *F*-test if ≤.05; ES (*d*), effect size for mean differences (treated vs. untreated) computed as Cohen's *d*.

Educational Therapies

Formal Academic Tutoring

Parents in the national survey also reported on the educational treatments their children had received. The results for all BSCTS-CA scores for those reporting that their children had received some type of formal academic tutoring outside of school are shown in Table 7.10. The initial MANOVA was significant (F = 16.35; df = 6,1915, $p < .001$). The univariate tests showed that children who had received tutoring had significantly higher scores on all of the BSCTS-CA scores (all *p*s < .001). Effect sizes for the SCT scores were in the medium range.

Special Educational Services

Children whose parents reported having received special education were compared to those who had not on all eight BSCTS-CA scores. The univariate tests showed that children who had received special education services in school had significantly higher scores on all of the BSCTS-CA SCT scores (all *p*s < .001). Effect sizes for SCT scores were in the medium range. As with formal tutoring, children receiving special educational services in school had significantly greater symptoms of SCT.

TABLE 7.10. Comparison of Children Who Had and Had Not Received Formal Academic Tutoring Outside of School on the BSCTS-CA SCT Subscale Scores

	No tutoring (N = 1,842)		Tutoring (N = 80)				
	Mean	*SD*	Mean	*SD*	*F*	*p*	ES (*d*)
SCT Daydreamy Score	6.2	2.2	8.2	4.2	59.38	<.001	0.60
SCT Sluggish Score	8.2	2.7	10.7	5.5	59.24	<.001	0.58
SCT Total Score	14.4	4.5	18.9	9.2	68.07	<.001	0.62
SCT Symptom Count Score	0.4	1.4	1.8	3.4	66.97	<.001	0.54

Note. F, results for the univariate *F*-test; *p*, probability value for the univariate *F*-test if ≤.05; ES (*d*), effect size for mean differences (treated vs. untreated) computed as Cohen's *d*.

TABLE 7.11. Comparison of Children Who Had and Had Not Received Special Educational Services in School on the BSCTS-CA SCT Subscale Scores

	No services (*N* = 1,746)		Special education (*N* = 176)				
	Mean	*SD*	Mean	*SD*	*F*	*p*	ES (*d*)
SCT Daydreamy Score	6.1	2.0	8.4	3.6	156.41	<.001	0.79
SCT Sluggish Score	8.0	2.5	10.8	4.6	176.84	<.001	0.76
SCT Total Score	14.1	4.3	19.2	7.5	191.24	<.001	0.83
SCT Symptom Count Score	0.3	1.3	1.8	2.9	148.55	<.001	0.67

Note. F, results for the univariate *F*-test; *p*, probability value for the univariate *F*-test if ≤.05; ES (*d*), effect size for mean differences (treated vs. untreated) computed as Cohen's *d*.

Speech and Language Therapy

As above, children who had received speech and language therapy at school ($N =$ 219) had significantly higher SCT scores on the BSCTS-CA than those who did not ($N = 1{,}703$) (all *p*s < .001). These results are not tabled for the sake of space.* Again, this is not surprising, given the finding in the previous chapter that children with language delays are more likely to have elevated SCT symptoms.

Occupational and Physical Therapy

Similar results to those for speech therapy were evident for those who had received occupational therapy services ($N = 85$) to those who had not ($N = 1{,}837$). Again, the results are not tabled here for the sake of saving space. Unlike ADHD, SCT has shown little if any evidence to date of an association with motor deficits. And precisely the same pattern of results was evident, not surprisingly, for children who had ($N = 58$) and had not ($N = 1{,}864$) received physical therapy.

Psychological Therapies

Parents reported that 187 children had received some type of individual psychological counseling or therapy. All univariate tests were significant at the $p < .001$ level, as shown in Table 7.12. Thus, children receiving individual psychological treatment are likely to have elevated SCT scores on the BSCTS-CA. Group differences for the SCT scores were of a medium magnitude. This same pattern held true for parents reporting that they had participated in family therapy ($N = 73$) (again, the results are not tabled to save space). In general, it appears that children receiving individual or family psychological treatment are likely to have elevations on SCT scores. The pattern of results for the small number of children who had participated in group therapy ($N = 18$) was that, again, all four scores were significantly elevated for SCT on the BSCTS-CA. Just 14 children had been placed in inpatient psychiatric

*Results for all untabled analyses reported in this manual are available upon request by writing to me—email: *drbarkley6769@comcast.net*—or through the website *www.russellbarkley.org*.

TABLE 7.12. Comparison of Children Who Had and Had Not Received Individual Psychological Treatment on the BSCTS-CA SCT Subscale Scores

	No therapy (*N* = 1,735)		Individual therapy (*N* = 187)				
	Mean	*SD*	Mean	*SD*	*F*	*p*	ES (*d*)
SCT Daydreamy Score	6.1	2.1	7.8	3.3	85.14	<.001	0.61
SCT Sluggish Score	8.1	2.6	10.2	4.7	98.74	<.001	0.55
SCT Total Score	14.2	4.4	18.0	7.5	106.51	<.001	0.62
SCT Symptom Count Score	0.3	1.3	1.4	2.7	81.52	<.001	0.52

Note. F, results for the univariate *F*-test; *p*, probability value for the univariate *F*-test if ≤.05; ES (*d*), effect size for mean differences (treated vs. untreated) computed as Cohen's *d*.

settings. The results for that group of children were identical in their pattern to that for those receiving group therapy.

Conclusions

The findings presented in this chapter provide varied and substantial evidence for the concurrent and ecological validity of the BSCTS-CA scores. It is clear here that BSCTS-CA scores are related to impairment in major life activities in each of the 15 domains of the BFIS-CA. Children having greater SCT symptoms are more likely to be rated by parents as being more impaired across all of these domains and as being impaired in more domains of life activities. This linkage of BSCTS-CA scores to impairment was also found in analyses of more specific areas of psychosocial impairment, such as community activities and sports participation, friendships and unpopularity, school adjustment (grades, retentions, suspensions/expulsions), and proneness to accidental injuries/poisonings. Higher scores on the BSCTS-CA were associated with greater risks across all of these domains to varying, yet significant, degrees. Differing patterns of subscale scores were also evident and were significantly associated with various forms of psychiatric, psychological, and educational treatments such that children placing in the clinically deficient range of the BSCTS-CA were significantly more likely to be receiving such services. Such findings make the BSCTS-CA the most validated parent rating scales of SCT in children that is currently available. All of these areas are clearly in need of more research, but what exists to date supports the validity of the scale for assessing SCT symptoms in daily life activities. Currently lacking and in need of more research is the sensitivity of the scale scores to various treatments recommended for the management of SCT. Nevertheless, the available evidence concerning validity supports the use of the BSCTS-CA in various clinical, scientific, educational, and other organizational settings where the assessment of SCT symptoms in the daily life of children is of interest.

CHAPTER 8

Scoring and Interpretation of the BSCTS-CA Forms

The BSCTS-CA can be used to evaluate attention deficits in the daily life activities of children ages 6–17 years. It can do so quickly and inexpensively in a clinical practice, research setting, or educational or organizational setting, among others. As with all of my other rating scales, the BSCTS-CA is intended for use by trained professionals in clinical, research, or educational/organizational specialties. Such professionals must have sufficient educational background and experience in the evaluation of child psychological functioning and its impairment. Interpretation of the BSCTS-CA scales, scores, and profiles requires graduate training in a psychological, psychiatric, educational, or medical specialty in which relevant graduate-level training and coursework have been obtained in the administration and interpretation of psychological measures through an accredited college or university. Besides carefully reviewing and understanding this manual, examiners using the BSCTS-CA should be familiar with the most recent version of the *Standards for Educational and Psychological Testing,* developed jointly by the American Educational Research Association, the American Psychological Association, and the American Council on Measurement in Education (2013).

BSCTS-CA Materials

The BSCTS-CA can be scored using one of four SCT Profiles, depending on the child's age group (6–11, 12–17) and sex, as provided in the Appendix. Raw scores corresponding to each subscale are computed from the BSCTS-CA scale and are then recorded on the bottom row of the Profile. One then looks up the corresponding column for that raw score and circles it. Then one can look to the far left- and right-hand columns to convert those raw scores in the columns to their respective percentiles from the national sample for the child's age group and sex.

Appropriate Purposes and Populations for the BSCTS-CA

The BSCTS-CA is not intended to replicate or replace the use of clinical interviews by professionals, relevant psychological testing, and other information needed to evaluate and diagnose children's attention disorders. Measures of impairment, such as archival records (school report cards, achievement tests, transcripts) and rating scales of functional effectiveness in major domains of children's life activities, such as the BFIS-CA (Barkley, 2012c), should also be collected to assess the consequences associated with the child's attention deficits in daily life.

The BSCTS-CA is intended as an evaluation tool of individuals between 6 and 17 years. The Barkley Adult ADHD Rating Scale–IV (BAARS-IV; Barkley, 2011a) can be used to evaluate this same attention disorder in adults' (ages 18–81 years) daily life activities. Typically, the children being evaluated will be those who reside in the United States because this country is the source for the normative sample. Use of the BSCTS-CA with populations, countries, cultures, or ethnic groups outside of the United States may be inappropriate to the extent that such groups may vary from the normative reference sample described in this manual.

Administration

The BSCTS-CA should be given directly to the parent whose child is being evaluated, along with a clear explanation of the purposes for which the rating scale is being obtained. The examiner should also provide a clear understanding of the instructions for completing the rating scale (see the Appendix) and an opportunity for the parent to have his/her concerns or questions about the scale addressed by the examiner. The BSCTS-CA may be mailed to parents to complete before the day of the intended evaluation, of which the BSCTS-CA is only a part. If that is the case, the scale should be accompanied by a cover letter that provides the above information concerning the purposes to which the scale is being put and the instructions for its completion. This letter should also contain a means by which the parent can contact the examiner about any concerns or questions he/she may have about the scale or its intended purpose.

The BSCTS-CA takes an average of approximately 5–10 minutes or less to complete by the average parent in the general population. After the form has been completed, review the scale for any missed items. Then encourage the rater to complete those items. The failure to complete more than a few items on the scale is likely to invalidate the resulting scores and make the use of the normative tables on the Profiles inappropriate. If the scale has been returned by mail and items are missing, have the parent complete them on the morning of the evaluation. If there is simply no further opportunity to get any missed items completed, then these items should be answered with a 1 (never or rarely) to create a conservative bias to the scores such that any attention problems are not unduly exaggerated. Even then, the failure to complete more than 5% of the items (2+) on the scale should be considered sufficient cause to invalidate the scale.

Scoring and Interpreting the BSCTS-CA

Scoring the BSCTS-CA Parent Rating Scale

Follow these procedures to score the BSCTS-CA:

- The easiest method for scoring is to start with Section 1. Add all of the answers circled in this section to get the total raw score. Write the answer in the line marked Section 1 Total Score in the shaded row at the end of this section marked "For Office Use Only."
- If you prefer, you can do this by an alternate means, as follows. Add all of the answers that are circled "1" (never or rarely) in column 2 of this section (the actual items or questions are in column 1). Place that sum in the empty box below that column (the box is in the shaded row marked "For Office Use Only"). Now do the same for column 3: Total all of the circled answers of "2s" (sometimes) in this column and place that sum at the bottom of that column in the empty box. Repeat this process for columns 4 (circled answers of often or 3s) and column 5 (very often or 4s). Now add these four sums together to get the total score for Section 1. Write the answer in the line marked Section 1 Total Score. Again, this will be in the shaded row at the end of this section. This is easier than it sounds here and takes less than 20–30 seconds to do per section.
- Repeat this same procedure for Section 2 (SCT Sluggish). These section scores correspond to each of the two subscales of the BSCTS-CA: Section 1 = SCT Daydreamy, and Section 2 = SCT Sluggish.
- When you have computed Sections 1 and 2 total scores, add them up to get the SCT Total Score; that is the total score for all items on the entire scale. Place the answer in the very last line of the scale marked "SCT Total Score" (this line is also shaded and marked "For Office Use Only").
- Finally, go back over Sections 1 and 2 for the SCT items and count the number of items that were answered with a 3 (often) or a 4 (very often) to get the SCT Symptom Count. Enter this number in the box so labeled in the last row of the scale, again marked "For Office Use Only."

You have now computed four scores for the BSCTS-CA: two for SCT, one for the SCT Total Score, and one for the SCT Symptom Counts (1).

At the end of Section 2, you will see the parents' answers to the questions about age of onset of the symptoms in these sections and whether these symptoms caused impairment (functional interference) in Home, Social, School, or Community domains. These answers are not scored for purposes of plotting them on the BSCTS-CA Profiles, but they can be transferred to the appropriate Profile for ease of interpreting the scale results. The DSM-5 requires that the age of onset for

ADHD symptoms leading to impairment must be 12 or younger. There is no such requirement for making a diagnosis of SCT because there are no official criteria for that disorder. Nevertheless, knowing the initial age of onset for SCT symptoms, as reported by parents, can be clinically informative.

Likewise, DSM-5 requires that symptoms of ADHD lead to impairment in one or more of these domains: Home, Social, School, or Community. Again, SCT has no official criterion for impairment. However, all disorders in DSM-5 require such a criterion, and SCT should be no exception. So, symptoms should be leading to impairment if an unofficial diagnosis of SCT is to be contemplated. In short, if the clinician finds that the child has sufficient symptoms of SCT to place in the clinical range (93rd percentile or higher) and has impairment in one or more of these four domains, then that child might meet criteria for an unofficial diagnosis of SCT.

Transferring Scores to the BSCTS-CA SCT Profiles

- Select the BSCTS-CA SCT Profile suitable for the child's age group and sex (ages 6–11 or 12–17 years, male or female) from the four Profiles provided in the Appendix.
- Up to four scores are possible to obtain from the scale, which will be plotted on this Profile. Transfer the raw scores you computed for each of the four sections of the BSCTS-CA scale into the appropriate cells in the very bottom row of that Profile; be sure to place the score in the appropriate column with the heading of the name of that score (e.g., SCT Daydreamy). Then transfer the raw scores from the last row of the rating scale that deal with the SCT Total Score and Symptom Count. Place these in the appropriate cells in the bottom row of the Profile.
- Each column that is related to the four raw scores, as provided on this Profile, shows a range of potential raw scores. Starting at the left-hand side of the Profile, under SCT Daydreamy, circle the raw score (or score range) in this column that reflects the respondent's raw score for Section 1 of the BSCTS-CA. That raw score is the number you transferred from the scale and recorded in the cell in the bottom row of the Profile.
- Look to the far left-hand column to determine the percentile of the general population that this score represents.
- Now do the same for the SCT Sluggish raw score (from Section 2 of the BSCTS-CA scale). Again, circle the score in this column that represents the raw score for Section 2 on the scale. Look to either the far left- or far right-hand column to see the percentile score associated with this raw score.
- Repeat this procedure for the SCT Total Score (the sum of the raw scores from Sections 1 and 2 related to all of the SCT items).
- Do this again for the SCT Symptom Count.
- To create a more visually obvious profile, you can draw lines that connect the circles you made around each raw score in each column. Start at the far left-hand side and draw a line connecting the circle in this column to the one in the next column, and so on, until you have lines connecting all the circles from left to right across the profile.

- The higher the percentile for any score, the more statistically deviant or abnormal is the score relative to the normative sample (general population). The percentiles that reflect the normal range of deficits are shown as ranges and then as individual percentiles starting at 70 and up to 99+. Raw scores are collapsed into ranges of scores at the lower percentiles for two reasons: (1) A large number of scores in the general population is found here, making the correspondence of each score to a single percentile difficult, if not impossible; and (2) scores in these lower percentile ranges generally have little clinical significance, other than to indicate that this individual is not elevated or abnormal in his/her level of attention deficits. However, scores in the highest quartile begin to spread out and take on some clinical significance as indicators of clinical deviancy and risks for impairments. For that reason, individual percentiles are provided for each raw score above the 70th percentile threshold.
- Generally, scores from the 76th to 84th percentile should be considered of *marginal* clinical significance. Those between the 85th and the 92rd percentiles would be considered *borderline or somewhat abnormal.* Those between the 93rd and 95th percentiles would be *mildly abnormal.* Those between the 96th and 98th percentiles would be considered *moderately abnormal.* And those at the 99th percentile would be viewed as *markedly abnormal or severe.*

Children who have a SCT Total Score or Symptom Count score that places at or above the 93rd percentile and who have impairment in at least one or more domains could be considered to be at high risk for an unofficial diagnosis of SCT.

BSCTS-CA Interview Form

Very rarely, situations may arise in which an individual being evaluated is unable to complete the BSCTS-CA, perhaps because he/she cannot read, cannot read English, or has a sufficiently severe visual impairment that precludes completing these rating scales. In these instances, the examiner may opt to use the BSCTS-CA Parent Interview, which is based on the BSCTS-CA items. It can also be found in the appendix. Examiners are strongly encouraged to use the BSCTS-CA rating scales whenever possible, as there are no norms that are directly applicable to the parent interview. But in these rare circumstances, the examiner can conduct a short interview with the parent using this BSCTS-CA Parent Interview form to determine if the child has significant deficits in these attention disorders in daily life activities.

Instructions to be read to the person being interviewed are provided at the top of the interview form. The individual is to be asked if his/her child has experienced each item during the past 6 months to a degree that is *often or very often* relative to other individuals in his/her age group. The examiner simply places a check in either the yes or no columns based on the response of the participant to each question. After the interview, the examiner adds up the number of yes responses to get the SCT Symptom Count. Although no norms are available for this interview form, it is likely that this score would be highly correlated with the BSCTS-CA rating scale Symptom Count Score. Therefore, to gain a very rough estimate of how deviant the parent reports are about a child on this interview, simply look at the column of raw scores on the SCT Profile for that child's age group and sex. Then look at the far left- or far right-hand column to note the percentile that corresponds to this raw score. Examiners must understand that this method provides only a very rough approximation of the status of this individual relative to others in the population using this Profile, because the interview form was not given to people in the normative sample. This is why examiners are encouraged to use the rating scale version of the BSCTS-CA whenever possible.

Evaluating Response to Treatment Using the BSCTS-CA

The BSCTS-CA can be a valuable tool in evaluating an individual's response to treatment, such as from cognitive training as part of neurorehabilitation interventions, CBT, or medication treatments.

How much change in a score would be needed to interpret that change as reliable? That is, how much change can be viewed as likely being the result of the intervention? Scientists and clinicians have employed various methods for determining how much change should be considered a positive (or negative) response to treatment, such as a change of 20, 30, or 40% from the baseline score. These, however, are quite arbitrary thresholds.

Instead, there are several statistical approaches for doing so that are better suited for this purpose. Unlike such arbitrarily defined thresholds for change, these statistical approaches take into consideration the test–retest reliability of the measure and the variation in change scores in the general population. Of these various approaches, one used quite frequently is the Reliable Change Index (RCI) developed by Jacobson (Jacobson & Truax, 1991; Jacobson, Roberts, Berns, & McGlinchey, 1999). This approach ensures that the degree of change exceeds that which may result merely from measurement error or unreliability. In essence, it shows if the change in the scores from pre- to posttreatment can be assumed, with 95% confidence (probability), to have come from a different distribution than that occurring as a consequence of variation and unreliability alone. A difference in scores of a magnitude at or exceeding the RCI number (threshold) would be expected less than 5% of the time by chance or unreliability of measurement alone.

The formula for calculating an RCI is $X_2 - X_1/S_{\text{diff}}$ where X_2 is the individual's posttest score and X_1 is his/her pretest score. The difference between the two is then divided by the standard error of the difference scores (S_{diff}). S_{diff} can be obtained directly from our results by using the standard deviations as well as the test–retest reliability information for each scale (Chapter 5), inserted into the formula above and as provided in the article by Jacobson and Truax (1991). The difference in means is divided by the S_{diff}. When the resultant number equals or exceeds 1.96, the difference is considered reliable (to occur 5% or less of the time by chance alone).

To save you time, the values of RCI needed to be considered a significant change on each subscale of the BSCTS-CA have been calculated for your convenience. To obtain these figures, I computed the S_{diff} for each scale and multiplied it by 1.96 to get the score needed to reach this threshold of significance. Those values are shown in Table 8.1 for each age group. To use them, simply take the posttest score of a patient or participant and subtract it from his/her pretest score. Then look in Table 8.1 for the row that corresponds to which subscale is being used to evaluate change. Look in the column of that row for the patient's age group. If this difference in the patient's scores exceeds the score in this cell of the table, then the change in pre- to posttest scores can be considered to be reliable, or outside the range of error of the measure. Probably the best score to use in these cases would be the SCT Total Scores, but the subscale scores of the BSCTS-CA can also be examined for their reliable change if that is of interest.

However, just because a change in scores is reliable does not necessarily make it clinically significant or meaningful. One means of determining such significance is to determine if the child now falls within the normal range following the intervention. That is, does the child's score after treatment allow one to conclude that it likely came from the normal range of scores in the general population? For this determination, Jacobson and Truax (1991) recommended that the posttreatment score now place within 2 *SD*s of the mean, or below the 98th percentile, for the normal population. This is a fairly generous interpretation of normalization. Others, such as myself, recommend that the posttreatment score place within 1.5 *SD*s of the normal mean, or approximately the 93rd percentile, since this is a threshold often used to determine if someone is clinically symptomatic or not. These demarcations for the general population sample for each age group are provided in Table 8.2. Thus, if a patient, following treatment, has shown (1) a change in scores from pretesting to posttesting that meets or surpasses the RCI score in Table 8.1 *and* (2) his/her final posttest score is within +1.5 *SD*s or +2 *SD*s of the mean for the normative sample (depending on how lenient the definition of recovery is chosen to be), as shown in Table 8.2, then one could conclude that the treatment had resulted not only in reliable change but also in recovery or normalization.

As an example, consider a male child within the age range of 6–11 years with ADHD or even a closed-head injury who is manifesting significant SCT symptoms in daily life, as reflected in an SCT Total Score from the BSCTS-CA of 46. Following the introduction of treatment for a month with an ADHD medication, the parent of this child completes the BSCTS-CA again, and now the child has an SCT Total Score of 14. Is this degree of change from the medication treatment reliable? That is, is it likely to fall outside the realm of merely measurement error or unreliability? To find out, compute the RCI as follows: Pretest score of 46 minus posttest score of

TABLE 8.1. The RCI Necessary for Pre- to Posttreatment Difference Scores to Be Significant (Reliable) on the Six Raw Scores from the BSCTS-CA Subscales

	RCI by age group and sex			
	6–11 years		12–17 years	
	Males	Females	Males	Females
SCT Daydreamy Score	3.09	2.92	3.18	2.79
SCT Sluggish Score	3.06	3.06	4.23	3.29
SCT Total Score	5.21	5.10	6.43	5.10

TABLE 8.2. The Thresholds for Determining Normalization or Recovery at Posttesting Following Treatment

	Age Group and Sex							
	6–11 years				12–17 years			
	Males		Females		Males		Females	
	+1.5	+2.0	+1.5	+2.0	+1.5	+2.0	+1.5	+2.0
SCT Daydreamy Score	9.8	11.0	9.6	10.8	10.2	11.5	9.6	10.7
SCT Sluggish Score	11.9	13.2	11.8	13.1	14.4	16.2	12.5	13.9
SCT Total Score	21.3	23.7	21.0	23.3	24.2	27.1	21.5	23.8

Note. Thresholds are provided for +1.5 and +2 *SD*s above the mean of the normative sample for each age group for the six BSCTS-CA raw scores.

14 = 32 points. Table 8.1 shows that for 6- to 11-year-old boys, the RCI needed to be significant for the SCT Total Score is 5.21. The patient's change score of 32 is above this RCI threshold. Thus, the clinician can feel confident that the improvement in ADHD symptoms is not simply due to measurement error or unreliability; rather, it is likely to be a consequence of the treatment. It is *reliable.* The patient could be considered as a treatment responder in this instance (assuming that side effects of the medication are not so annoying as to warrant treatment discontinuation).

Next we wish to know if the child has been normalized by the treatment—that is, has the intervention brought him/her to within the normal range. Examine Table 8.2 to see that the threshold of +2 *SD*s above the normal mean for boys who are 6–11 years is 23, which corresponds to approximately the 98th percentile. The patient's posttest score of 14 is well below this figure, and so could be considered to place within the broadly defined normal range. However, as noted above, some clinicians and researchers (such as myself) believe that this is too generous a definition of normalcy for determining recovery. Using the criterion of +1.5 *SD*s above the normal mean may be preferred. In that case, checking the appropriate column of Table 8.2, we find that this threshold is 21. The patient's posttest score of 14 is also below this level. And so, even by this more conservative definition of normalization, the patient can be considered to place within the broadly defined normal range for his/her age group and sex following treatment. This score may be considered to indicate "recovery." By this empirical approach to defining a treatment responder (RCI) and normalization, the treatment has been successful.

Of course, ADHD medications provide only symptomatic relief in such cases and only when the medication is taken at therapeutic levels. Therefore, the resulting reliable change (positive response) and normalization refer only to a temporary effect of the medication while in use and not to a permanent alteration of the patient's functioning in the absence of medication management.

To add further to the utility of such an evaluation of an ADHD medication, a clinician might want to have the parent complete the Side Effects Questionnaire (Barkley & Murphy, 2006) both before and after treatment. This is done to ensure that the changes taking place in any reported adverse events are, in fact, a consequence of the medication and not merely preexisting conditions that went unexamined prior to the medication trial.

Evaluating Change in SCT Due to Brain Injury

A very similar approach can be taken to evaluating whether or not a child or teen has experienced a significant deterioration in his/her attention in daily life activities following some form of brain injury, whether the origin is from a traumatic, infectious, cancerous, or vascular event or other causal factor. In this case, the clinician here may be asking the question, "Has a reliable and significant decline in attention in daily life occurred in this patient?" The RCI figures in Table 8.1 can be used to determine if the deterioration in functioning is reliable (probably outside the realm of measurement error). The parent can complete the BSCTS-CA on how he/she believes the child is functioning now. Next, the parent can complete a second version with reference to how well he/she believes the child was functioning prior to the event. Then the clinician can compare the patient's premorbid and postmorbid SCT Total Scores.

Once again, to get the RCI, subtract the postmorbid from the premorbid score, which in this case will be negative. Now look in Table 8.1 for the SCT Total Score for the patient's age group and sex. If the difference in the patient's scores is higher than the one in the table, the patient's deterioration in functioning, as found on the BSCTS-CA, can be considered to be reliable—that is, the change is probably outside the realm of measurement error or unreliability (likely to occur 5% or less of the time). The thresholds provided in Table 8.2 for the child's age group and sex and this BSCTS-CA score can now be used to determine if the child's scores now place him/her *outside* of the normal range, using both the +1.5 *SD* and +2 *SD* thresholds (approximately the 93rd and 98th percentiles). That is to say that the child's postmorbid score is now more likely to have been drawn from a distribution of individuals impaired or disordered in their attention in daily life activities than to have been drawn from the general adult population.

Interpreting the BSCTS-CA

The professional interpretation of the results of the BSCTS-CA begins with the examiner's thorough understanding of the nature of this attention disorder, as described in Chapter 1. Yet the chapter is not a substitute for a more thorough grounding in the larger literature on these conditions, though it will suffice for SCT at the moment, given the small quantity of literature on that condition. It is therefore essential that the examiner have not only a thorough understanding of the earlier chapters of this manual, but also familiarity with the literature on SCT, especially as SCT is manifested in daily life activities.

Further interpretation of the scale is based on the following approaches to understanding the meaning of the scores.

Face Validity

This approach to interpretation is aided by a complete familiarity with the items contained on the scale and the four sections (subscales) to which those items have been assigned. High scores on each subscale or the total scores of the subscales (typically at or above the 93rd percentile and especially at or above the 98th) may signal the existence of an attention disorder as it occurs in daily life activities. One initial means of interpreting each scale in a clinical report is on the basis of the face validity of that subscale. The examiner can actually interpret the meaning of the scale score from the name given to that scale (e.g., SCT Daydreamy). This interpretation can be enhanced by selecting the individual items from that subscale on which the respondent has answered a 3 or 4 (a symptom) and directly quoting these items in that portion of the report to convey the meaning of that scale. Given that the scales are moderately intercorrelated, it is possible that an individual will obtain abnormal scores in SCT subscales of the BSCTS-CA, yet it is just as possible that only one or the other will be clinically elevated. Also, in view of this interrelatedness of the scales, computing interscale differences is not encouraged because the meaning of disparities across the scales has not been explored in any research to date. This does not mean, however, that relative fluctuations across the scales will not be evident—only that interpreting the meaning of large disparities between scales has no empirical basis at this time. Just interpreting the meaning of each scale separately is likely to be sufficient to convey the meaning of the BSCTS-CA scores, rather than trying to torture the score comparisons to yield up more information than exists about them at the present time.

Normative Comparison

Further interpretation of each subscale score continues with the comparison of the individual's scores to that of the normative population using the SCT Profiles and the resulting percentiles so obtained for them in the Appendix. This is then reported as the relative position of the individual in comparison to the general population of children/adolescents, specifically to the age group and sex of the child, and the norms used to obtain the percentile score. In short, using the percentile score, the individual is said to place at or above this percentage of individuals in the general population of his/her age group and sex in the manifestation of these attention disorders in daily life activities.

Risk Analysis (Using the Evidence on Criterion or Predictive Validity)

As discussed in Chapters 6 and 7, high scores on the BSCTS-CA subscales were associated with a variety of psychiatric disorders, risks for various treatments, and other difficulties in various domains of major life activities. Therefore, the higher the scores observed on the BSCTS-CA, the more likely is the child to be at risk for problems in these same domains of life activities. These risks should be noted in the clinical interpretation of the larger meaning of the BSCTS-CA scores beyond their simply reflecting the SCT symptoms for which the subscales are named. Problems with educational, family, peer, and community functioning, and various forms of psychological distress or psychiatric disorders (anxiety, depression, etc.) were all correlates of higher BSCTS-CA scores that deserve notice by the examiner and probably should be conveyed to the parent when appropriate and applicable. Such information can also be linked to what is already known about the child from the larger evaluation in which the BSCTS-CA should serve as simply one component when used for a clinical evaluation of a patient. The examiner will have information on the history of the child with regard to these and other major domains of life activity that can serve to place the findings from the BSCTS-CA in this larger context. The BSCTS-CA results can perhaps provide additional hypotheses or even explanations as to why adverse events in these various life domains may have been a consequence of, or at least related to, deficits associated with SCT. This risk analysis concerning impairments can be further aided by using the BFIS-CA (Barkley, 2012b), for which national norms are available for parent ratings of potential impairment in 15 major domains of children's daily life activities.

Pre–Postinjury Changes

As already noted above, another approach to interpreting the BSCTS-CA exists when the scale has been used to assess possible changes in an individual secondary to a neurological injury, or in conjunction with the onset of an acute adverse psychiatric or psychological event. If the BSCTS-CA was given twice to a parent of a pediatric patient with instructions to complete one version for preinjury status and the other for postinjury, then these comparisons can be interpreted, with appropriate caution, based on the information they may provide on the impact of the event on SCT symptoms in daily life activities. Obviously the caveat that these ratings are from parent recall and were not collected pre- and postinjury needs to be noted in discussing such results.

Pre–Posttreatment

As discussed above, the BSCTS-CA can also be used to evaluate possible response to intervention by giving the scale to parents before and after an intervention has been implemented with their child. Guidelines were given above and in Tables 8.1 and 8.2 for how to interpret a change in scores as reflecting reliable change and recovery or normalization. This information can be included in the interpretation of the meaning of the BSCTS-CA scores so obtained.

Conclusions

The BSCTS-CA provides a clinically informative means of evaluating SCT symptoms as reported by parents in the daily life activities of their children, ages 6–17 years. Further research on and clinical experience with the BSCTS-CA is strongly encouraged. Meanwhile, evidence to date shows the BSCTS-CA to be reasonably reliable, valid, and useful in assessing these dimensions of attention disorders in the daily life activities of children and teenagers. It does so by a means that is efficient and cost-effective. It also yields valuable information on the potential risks that such deficits may be posing in the extent to which the symptoms of these two attention disorders may relate to potential impairments in a variety of domains of major life activities. The adaptive meaningfulness of the BSCTS-CA is documented in its association with impairment in a variety of domains of major life activities for children and adolescents, beyond simply documenting the existence of such an attention disorder and its symptoms. The scale can be used in clinical practice, in research and educational/organization settings, and in other such venues where the evaluation of SCT symptoms in the daily life activities of children or teenagers is of interest. It can also serve as a basis for evaluating change in such an attention disorder whether as a consequence of treatment or secondary to the occurrence of various neurological and psychiatric disorders, or even transient psychological events believed to potentially impact a child's attention performance adversely in daily life activities. As with the adult version of this scale, I hope that you find these scales useful in your practice.

APPENDIX

BSCTS-CA Forms and SCT Profiles

BSCTS-CA Parent Rating Scale

Child's name: ______________________________ Date: ______________

Child's Sex: Male ____ Female ____ Child's age (in years): ______________

Child's grade in school (K to 12): ______

Is this your biological child? Yes ____ No ____

Your relationship to this child: Mother ____ Father ____ Stepmother ____ Stepfather ____
Adoptive mother ____ Adoptive father ____ Other (specify): ______________

Your age (in years): ______________ Your education (in years): ______________

Other parent's age (in years): ______________ Other parent's education (in years): ______________

Instructions

How often does this child experience each of these problems? Please circle the number next to each item that best describes his/her behavior **DURING THE PAST 6 MONTHS.** If your child is currently taking medication for any psychiatric or psychological disorder, please rate his/her behavior based on how he/she acts while **OFF** the medication. Ignore the shaded boxes below marked "For Office Use Only."

Section 1	Never or rarely	Sometimes	Often	Very often
D1. Prone to daydreaming	1	2	3	4
D2. Mentally foggy or easily confused	1	2	3	4
D3. Stares a lot	1	2	3	4
D4. Spacey; his/her mind seems to be elsewhere and not paying attention to what is going on around him/her	1	2	3	4
D5. Gets lost in his/her thoughts	1	2	3	4
For Office Use Only: **Section 1 Total Score** ________				
Section 2	Never or rarely	Sometimes	Often	Very often
1. Has trouble staying alert or awake	1	2	3	4
2. Lethargic, more tired than others or lacks energy	1	2	3	4
3. Underactive compared to other children	1	2	3	4
4. Slow moving or sluggish	1	2	3	4
5. Doesn't seem to understand or process questions or explanations as quickly or as accurately as others	1	2	3	4
6. Seems drowsy, or has a sleepy appearance	1	2	3	4
7. Apathetic or withdrawn; seems less engaged in activities than others	1	2	3	4

(continued)

8. If you answered 3 (Often) or 4 (Very often) to any of the items in Sections 1 and 2, at what age did you first notice these symptoms?		
9. If you answered 3 (Often) or 4 (Very often) to any of the items in Sections 1 and 2, do any of them interfere with your child's ability to function effectively in any of the following situations? (Circle No or Yes after each item.)		
9a. Home life with family	No	Yes
9b. Social relations with other children	No	Yes
9c. School	No	Yes
9d. Community activities (church, clubs, scouts, etc.)	No	Yes
For Office Use Only: **Section 2 Total Score** ______		
Sum of totals from Sections 1 and 2 for the SCT Total Score ______ **SCT Symptom Count** ______ **[The Symptom Count is the number of answers of 3 (Often) or 4 (Very often) in Sections 1 and 2.]**		

BSCTS-CA Parent Interview

Child's name: ______________________________ Date: ______________

Child's sex: Male ____ Female ____ Age: ______________

Name of person completing this form: ______________________________

Relationship to this child: Mother ____ Father ____ Stepmother ____ Stepfather ____
Other (specify): ______________________________

Instructions to Interviewer

Say the following to the person to be interviewed: "I would like to ask you a number of questions about your child's behavior during the past 6 months. For each behavior I ask you about, I want to know if it occurs often or more frequently."

Place a check mark (✓) in the box after each item indicating the answer of the person being interviewed. Each item is simply answered Yes or No.

SCT Questions	No, this does not occur often	Yes, this occurs often or very often
1. Prone to daydreaming		
2. Mentally foggy or easily confused		
3. Stares a lot		
4. Spacey; his/her mind seems to be elsewhere and not paying attention to what is going on around him/her		
5. Gets lost in his/her thoughts		
6. Has trouble staying alert or awake		
7. Lethargic, more tired than others or lacks energy		
8. Underactive compared to other children		
9. Slow moving or sluggish		
10. Doesn't seem to understand or process questions or explanations as quickly or as accurately as others		
11. Seems drowsy, or has a sleepy appearance		
12. Apathetic or withdrawn; seems less engaged in activities than others		
[EXAMINER: If the parent answered Yes to any of the above items, ask the following question.] Please tell me at what age those difficulties began (age in years). ________		

(continued)

[EXAMINER: If the parent answered Yes to any of the above items, ask the following question.] Please tell me if any of these behaviors interfered with your child's ability to function effectively in any of the following situations. Then circle "No" or "Yes" next to each domain of life.		
Home life with family	No	Yes
Social relations with other children	No	Yes
School	No	Yes
Community activities (church, clubs, Scouts, etc.)	No	Yes
For Office Use Only: **SCT Symptom Count** _______ **[Number of Yes answers to questions 1–12 on the previous page]**		

BSCTS-CA SCT Profile (Ages 6–11, Males Only)

Name: ______________________ Age: ______ Sex: ______ Date: ____________

Raw Scores and Percentiles for Each Subscale

%	SCT Daydreamy	SCT Sluggish	SCT Total Score	SCT Symptom Count	%
99+	18–20	21–28	33–48	7–12	99+
98	13–15	15–19	27–32	5–6	98
97	—	14	26	4	97
96	12	—	24–25	3	96
95	11	—	—	2	95
94	10	13	—	—	94
93	—	12	23	—	93
92	—	11	22	1	92
91	—	—	20–21	—	91
90	9	10	19	—	90
89	—	—	18	—	89
88	—	—	—	—	88
87	8	9	17	—	87
86	—	—	—	0	86
85	—	—	—	—	85
84	7	—	16	—	84
83	—	—	—	—	83
82	—	—	—	—	82
81	—	8	—	—	81
80	—	—	15	—	80
79	—	—	—	—	79

Sample size = 451

(continued)

BSCTS-CA SCT Profile (Ages 6–11, Males Only) *(page 2 of 2)*

%	SCT Daydreamy	SCT Sluggish	SCT Total Score	SCT Symptom Count	%
78	—	—	—	—	78
77	—	—	14	—	77
76	6	—	—	—	76
75	—	—	—	—	75
74	—	—	—	—	74
73	—	—	—	—	73
72	—	—	—	—	72
71	—	7	—	—	71
70	—	—	—	—	70
60–69	—	—	13	—	60–69
50–59	—	—	12	—	50–59
40–49	—	—	—	—	40–49
30–39	—	—	—	—	30–39
20–29	—	—	—	—	20–29
10–19	—	—	—	—	10–19
1–9	5	—	—	—	1–9
Raw Score from scale					Raw Score from scale

BSCTS-CA SCT Profile (Ages 6–11, Females Only)

Name: ______________________ Age: ______ Sex: ______ Date: ____________

Raw Scores and Percentiles for Each Subscale

%	SCT Daydreamy	SCT Sluggish	SCT Total Score	SCT Symptom Count	%
99+	16–20	21–28	35–48	8–12	99+
98	14–15	16–20	27–34	4–7	98
97	12–13	14–15	25–26	—	97
96	11	—	24	3	96
95	10	13	23	2	95
94	—	12	22	1	94
93	—	11	21	—	93
92	—	—	19–20	—	92
91	9	10	—	—	91
90	—	—	18	—	90
89	—	9	—	0	89
88	8	—	17	—	88
87	—	8	—	—	87
86	—	—	16	—	86
85	—	—	—	—	85
84	7	—	15	—	84
83	—	—	—	—	83
82	—	—	—	—	82
81	—	—	—	—	81
80	—	—	—	—	80
79	—	—	14	—	79

Sample size = 451

(continued)

BSCTS-CA SCT Profile (Ages 6–11, Females Only) *(page 2 of 2)*

%	SCT Daydreamy	SCT Sluggish	SCT Total Score	SCT Symptom Count	%
78	—	—	—	—	78
77	—	—	—	—	77
76	6	—	—	—	76
75	—	7	—	—	75
74	—	—	—	—	74
73	—	—	—	—	73
72	—	—	—	—	72
71	—	—	—	—	71
70	—	—	—	—	70
60–69	—	—	13	—	60–69
50–59	5	—	12	—	50–59
40–49	—	—	—	—	40–49
30–39	—	—	—	—	30–39
20–29	—	—	—	—	20–29
10–19	—	—	—	—	10–19
1–9	—	—	—	—	1–9
Raw Score from scale					Raw Score from scale

BSCTS-CA SCT Profile (Ages 12–17, Males Only)

Name: ______________________ Age: ______ Sex: ______ Date: ____________

Raw Scores and Percentiles for Each Subscale

%	SCT Daydreamy	SCT Sluggish	SCT Total Score	SCT Symptom Count	%
99+	17–20	22–28	39–48	11–12	99+
98	15–16	20–21	35–38	9–10	98
97	14	19	32–34	7–8	97
96	13	18	28–31	5–6	96
95	12	17	27	—	95
94	11	15–16	26	4	94
93	10	14	25	3	93
92	—	—	24	—	92
91	—	—	—	2	91
90	—	—	—	—	90
89	—	—	22–23	—	89
88	9	—	—	1	88
87	—	—	21	—	87
86	—	13	—	—	86
85	8	12	20	—	85
84	—	—	—	—	84
83	—	11	19	—	83
82	—	—	18	—	82
81	—	10	—	0	81
80	—	—	—	—	80
79	—	—	17	—	79

Sample size = 450

(continued)

BSCTS-CA SCT Profile (Ages 12–17, Males Only) *(page 2 of 2)*

%	SCT Daydreamy	SCT Sluggish	SCT Total Score	SCT Symptom Count	%
78	—	—	—	—	78
77	7	—	—	—	77
76	—	—	16	—	76
75	—	—	—	—	75
74	—	—	—	—	74
73	—	—	—	—	73
72	—	—	—	—	72
71	—	—	—	—	71
70	—	8–9	15	—	70
60–69	6	—	14	—	60–69
50–59	5	7	13	—	50–59
40–49	—	—	12	—	40–49
30–39	—	—	—	—	30–39
20–29	—	—	—	—	20–29
10–19	—	—	—	—	10–19
1–9	—	—	—	—	1–9
Raw Score from scale					Raw Score from scale

BSCTS-CA SCT Profile (Ages 12–17, Females Only)

Name: ______________________ Age: ______ Sex: ______ Date: ____________

Raw Scores and Percentiles for Each Subscale

%	SCT Daydreamy	SCT Sluggish	SCT Total Score	SCT Symptom Count	%
99+	15–20	20–28	31–48	7–12	99+
98	13–14	17–19	28–30	6	98
97	12	15–16	26–27	4–5	97
96	11	—	24–25	3	96
95	10	14	—	—	95
94	—	—	23	2	94
93	—	13	22	—	93
92	9	12	21	1	92
91	—	—	—	—	91
90	—	—	20	—	90
89	—	11	—	—	89
88	—	—	—	—	88
87	8	—	18–19	—	87
86	—	10	—	0	86
85	—	—	—	—	85
84	—	—	17	—	84
83	—	9	—	—	83
82	—	—	—	—	82
81	7	—	—	—	81
80	—	—	16	—	80
79	—	—	—	—	79

Sample size = 448

(continued)

BSCTS-CA SCT Profile (Ages 12–17, Females Only) *(page 2 of 2)*

%	SCT Daydreamy	SCT Sluggish	SCT Total Score	SCT Symptom Count	%
78	—	—	—	—	78
77	—	—	—	—	77
76	—	8	15	—	76
75	—	—	—	—	75
74	—	—	—	—	74
73	—	—	—	—	73
72	—	—	—	—	72
71	6	—	—	—	71
70	—	—	14	—	70
60–69	—	7	13	—	60–69
50–59	5	—	12	—	50–59
40–49	—	—	—	—	40–49
30–39	—	—	—	—	30–39
20–29	—	—	—	—	20–29
10–19	—	—	—	—	10–19
1–9	—	—	—	—	1–9
Raw Score from scale					Raw Score from scale

References

Abikoff, H. (1985). Efficacy of cognitive training interventions in hyperactive children: A critical review. *Clinical Psychology Review, 5,* 479–512.

Achenbach, T. M. (2001). *Manual for the Child Behavior Checklist/4–18 and 1991 Profile.* Burlington, VT: Author.

Achenbach, T. M., McConaughy, S. H., & Howell, C. T. (1987). Child/adolescent behavioral and emotional problems: Implications of cross-informant correlations for situational specificity. *Psychological Bulletin, 101,* 213–232.

Adams, Z. W., Milich, R., & Fillmore, M. T. (2010). A case for the return of attention-deficit disorder in DSM-5. *The ADHD Report, 18*(3), 1–6.

American Educational Research Association, American Psychological Association, & American Council on Measurement in Education. (2013). *Standards for educational and psychological testing.* Washington, DC: American Educational Research Association.

American Psychiatric Association. (1980). *Diagnostic and statistical manual of mental disorders* (3rd ed.). Washington, DC: Author.

American Psychiatric Association. (1987). *Diagnostic and statistical manual of mental disorders* (3rd ed., rev.). Washington, DC: Author.

American Psychiatric Association. (1994). *Diagnostic and statistical manual of mental disorders* (4th ed.). Washington, DC: Author.

American Psychiatric Association. (2000). *Diagnostic and statistical manual of mental disorders* (4th ed., text rev.). Washington, DC: Author.

American Psychiatric Association. (2013). *Diagnostic and statistical manual of mental disorders* (5th ed.). Arlington, VA: Author.

Angold, A., Costello, E. J., & Erkanli, A. (1999). Comorbidity. *Journal of Child Psychology and Psychiatry, 40,* 57–88.

Antshel, K. M., & Remer, R. (2003). Social skills training in children with attention deficit hyperactivity disorder: A randomized-controlled clinical trial. *Journal of Clinical Child and Adolescent Psychology, 32,* 153–165.

Barkley, R. A. (2011a). *Barkley Adult ADHD Rating Scale—IV (BAARS-IV).* New York: Guilford Press.

Barkley, R. A. (2011b). *Barkley Functional Impairment Scale (BFIS)*. New York: Guilford Press.

Barkley, R. A. (2011c). *Barkley Deficits in Executive Functioning Scale (BDEFS)*. New York: Guilford Press.

Barkley, R. A. (2012a). Distinguishing sluggish cognitive tempo from attention deficit hyperactivity disorder in adults. *Journal of Abnormal Psychology, 121,* 978–990.

Barkley, R. A. (2012b). *Executive functions: What they are, how they work, and why they evolved.* New York: Guilford Press.

Barkley, R. A. (2012c). *Barkley Functional Impairment Scale—Children and Adolescents (BFIS-CA)*. New York: Guilford Press.

Barkley, R. A. (2012d). *The Barkley Deficits in Executive Functioning Scale—Children and Adolescents (BDEFS-CA)*. New York: Guilford Press.

Barkley, R. A. (2013). Distinguishing sluggish cognitive tempo from ADHD in children and adolescents: Executive functioning, impairment, and comorbidity. *Journal of Clinical Child and Adolescent Psychology, 42,* 161–173.

Barkley, R. A. (2014). Sluggish cognitive tempo (concentration deficit disorder?): Current status, future directions, and a plea to change the name. *Journal of Abnormal Child Psychology, 42,* 117–125.

Barkley, R. A. (2015a). Concentration deficit disorder (sluggish cognitive tempo). In R. A. Barkley (Ed.), *Attention-deficit hyperactivity disorder: A handbook for diagnosis and treatment* (4th ed., pp. 435–454). New York: Guilford Press.

Barkley, R. A. (2015b). Executive functioning and self-regulation viewed as an extended phenotype: Implications of the theory for ADHD and its treatment. In R. A. Barkley (Ed.), *Attention-deficit hyperactivity disorder: A handbook for diagnosis and treatment* (4th ed., pp. 405–434). New York: Guilford Press.

Barkley, R. A. (2015c). Health problems and related impairments in children and adults. In R. A. Barkley (Ed.), *Attention-deficit hyperactivity disorder: A handbook for diagnosis and treatment* (4th ed., pp. 267–313). New York: Guilford Press.

Barkley, R. A., DuPaul, G. J., & McMurray, M. B. (1991). Attention deficit disorder with and without hyperactivity: Clinical response to three doses of methylphenidate. *Pediatrics, 87,* 519–531.

Barkley, R. A., & Fischer, M. (2011). Predicting impairment in major life activities and occupational functioning in hyperactive children as adults: Self-reported executive function (EF) deficits vs. EF tests. *Developmental Neuropsychology, 36*(2), 137–161.

Barkley, R. A., & Murphy, K. R. (2006). *Attention-deficit hyperactivity disorder: A clinical workbook* (3rd ed.). New York: Guilford Press.

Barkley, R. A., & Murphy, K. R. (2010). Impairment in occupational functioning and adult ADHD: The predictive utility of executive function (EF) ratings vs. EF tests. *Archives of Clinical Neuropsychology, 25,* 157–173.

Barkley, R. A., Murphy, K. R., & Fischer, M. (2008). *ADHD in adults: What the science says.* New York: Guilford Press.

Bauermeister, J. J., Barkley, R. A., Bauermeister, J. A., Martinez, J. V., & McBurnett, K. (2012). Validity of the sluggish cognitive tempo, inattention, and hyperactivity symptom dimensions: Neuropsychological and psychosocial correlates. *Journal of Abnormal Child Psychology, 40,* 683–697.

Becker, S. P., Burns, G. L., Garner, A. A., Jarrett, M. A., Luebbe, A. M., Epstein, J. N., et al. (2017, July 13). Sluggish cognitive tempo in adults: Psychometric validation of the Adult Concentration Inventory. *Psychological Assessment.* Epub ahead of print.

Becker, S. P., Burns, G. L., Schmitt, A. P., Epstein, J. N., & Tamm, L. (2017). Toward establishing a standard symptom set for assessing sluggish cognitive tempo in children: Evidence from teacher ratings in a community sample. *Assessment.* Epub ahead of print.

Becker, S. P., Garner, A. A., & Byars, K. C. (2016). Sluggish cognitive tempo in children referred to a pediatric Sleep Disorders Center: Examining possible overlap with sleep problems and associations with impairment. *Journal of Psychiatric Research, 77,* 116–124.

Becker, S. P., & Langberg, J. M. (2013). Sluggish cognitive tempo among young adolescents with ADHD: Relations to mental health, academic, and social functioning. *Journal of Attention Disorders, 17*(8), 681–689.

Becker, S. P., & Langberg, J. M. (2014). Attention-deficit/hyperactivity disorder and sluggish cognitive tempo dimensions in relation to executive functioning in adolescents with ADHD. *Child Psychiatry and Human Development, 45*(1), 1–11.

Becker, S. P., Langberg, J. M., Luebbe, A. M., Dvorsky, M. R., & Flannery, A. J. (2014). Sluggish cognitive tempo is associated with academic functioning and internalizing symptoms in college students with and without attention-deficit/hyperactivity disorder. *Journal of Clinical Psychology, 70,* 388–403.

Becker, S. P., Leopold, D. R., Burns, G. L., Jarrett, M. A., Langberg, J. M., Marshall, S. A., et al. (2016). Internal, external, and diagnostic validity of sluggish cognitive tempo: A meta-analysis and critical review. *Journal of the American Academy of Child and Adolescent Psychiatry, 55,* 163–178.

Becker, S. P., Luebbe, A. M., Fite, P. J., Stoppelbein, L., & Greening, L. (2014). Sluggish cognitive tempo in psychiatrically hospitalized children: Factor structure and relations to internalizing symptoms, social problems, and observed behavioral dysregulation. *Journal of Abnormal Child Psychology, 42*(1), 49–62.

Becker, S. P., Luebbe, A. M., & Langberg, J. M. (2014). Attention-deficit/hyperactivity disorder dimensions and sluggish cognitive tempo symptoms in relation to college students' sleep functioning. *Child Psychiatry and Human Development, 45,* 675–685.

Belmar, M., Servera, M., Becker, S. P., & Burns, G. L. (2015). Validity of sluggish cognitive tempo in South America: An initial examination using mother and teacher ratings of Chilean children. *Journal of Attention Disorders, 21,* 667–672.

Biederman, J., Petty, C. R., Fried, R., Black, S., Faneuil, A., Doyle, A. E., et al. (2008). Discordance between psychometric testing and questionnaire-based definitions of executive function deficits in individuals with ADHD. *Journal of Attention Disorders, 12,* 92–102.

Boyle, C. A., Decoufle, P., & Yeargin-Allsop, M. (1994). Prevalence and health impact of developmental disabilities in U.S, children. *Pediatrics, 93,* 399–403.

Brandenburg, N. A., Friedman, R. M., & Silver, S. E. (1990). The epidemiology of childhood psychiatric disorders: Prevalence findings from recent studies. *Journal of the American Academy of Child and Adolescent Psychiatry, 29,* 76–83.

Brown, T. E. (Ed.). (2009). *ADHD comorbidities: Handbook for ADHD complications in children and adults.* Arlington, VA: American Psychiatric Association Publishing.

Bryant, F. B. (2000). Assessing the validity of measurement. In. L. G. Grim & P. R. Yarnold (Eds.), *Reading and understanding more multivariate statistics* (pp. 99–146). Washington, DC: American Psychological Association.

Burns, C. L., Servera, M., Bernad, M. M., Carrillo, J. M., & Cardo, E. (2013). Distinctions between sluggish cognitive tempo, ADHD-IN, and depression symptom dimensions in Spanish first-grade children. *Journal of Clinical Child and Adolescent Psychology, 42,* 796–808.

Camprodon-Rosanas, E., Batlle, S., Estrada-Prat, X., Aceña-Diaz, M., Petrizan-Aleman, A., Pujals, E., et al. (2016). Sluggish cognitive tempo in child and adolescent clinical outpatient setting. *Journal of Psychiatric Practice, 22,* 355–362.

Camprodon-Rosanas, E., Ribas-Fitó, N., Batlle, S., Persavento, C., Alvarexz-Pedrerol, M., Sunyer, J., et al. (2017a, April 1). Association between sluggish cognitive tempo symptoms and attentional network and working memory in primary schoolchildren. *Journal of Attention Disorders.* Epub ahead of print.

Camprodon-Rosanas, E., Ribas-Fitó, N., Batlle-Vila, S., Persavento, C., Alvarexz-Pedrerol,

M., Sunyer, J., et al. (2017b). Sluggish cognitive tempo: Sociodemographic, behavioral, and clinical characteristics in a population of Catalan school children. *Journal of Attention Disorders, 21,* 632–641.

Capdevila-Brophy, C., Artigas-Pallares, J., Nacarro-Pastor, J. B., Garcia-Nonell, K., Rigau-Ratera, E., & Obiols, J. E. (2012). ADHD predominantly inattentive subtype with high sluggish cognitive tempo: A new clinical entity? *Journal of Attention Disorders, 18,* 607–616.

Carlson, C. L. (1986). Attention deficit disorder with and without hyperactivity: A review of preliminary experimental evidence. In B. B. Lahey & A. E. Kazdin (Eds.), *Advances in clinical child psychology* (Vol. 9, pp. 153–175). New York: Plenum Press.

Carlson, C. L., Lahey, B. B., & Neeper, R. (1986). Direct assessment of the cognitive correlates of attention deficit disorders with and without hyperactivity. *Journal of Behavioral Assessment and Psychopathology, 8,* 69–86.

Carlson, C. L., & Mann, M. (2002). Sluggish cognitive tempo predicts a different pattern of impairment in the attention deficit hyperactivity disorder, predominantly inattentive type. *Journal of Clinical Child and Adolescent Psychology, 31,* 123–129.

Christoff, K., Irving, Z. C., Fox, K. C. R., Spreng, N., & Andrews-Hanna, A. (2016). Mind-wandering as spontaneous thought: A dynamic framework. *Nature Reviews Neuroscience, 17,* 718–731.

Cohen, J. (1992). A power primer. *Psychological Bulletin, 112,* 155–159.

Combs, M. A., Canu, W. H., Broman, J. J., & Nieman, D. C. (2013). Impact of sluggish cognitive tempo and attention-deficit/hyperactivity disorder symptoms on adults' quality of life. *Applied Research in Quality of Life, 9,* 981–995.

Combs, M. A., Canu, W. H., Broman-Fulks, J. J., Rocheleau, C. A., & Nieman, D. C. (2012). Perceived stress and ADHD symptoms in adults. *Journal of Attention Disorders, 19,* 425–434.

Cook, T. D., & Campbell, D. T. (1979). *Quasi-experimentation: Design and analysis issues for field settings.* Chicago: Rand McNally.

Costello, E. J., Egger, H., & Angold, A. (2005). 10-year research update review: The epidemiology of child and adolescent psychiatric disorders: I. Methods and public health burden. *Journal of the American Academy of Child and Adolescent Psychiatry, 44,* 972–986.

Costello, E. J., Mustillo, S., Erkanli, A., Keeler, G., & Angold, A. (2003). Prevalence and development of psychiatric disorders in childhood and adolescence. *Archives of General Psychiatry, 60,* 837–844.

Crichton, A. (1976). *An inquiry into the nature and origin of mental derangement: comprehending a concise system of the physiology and pathology of the human mind and a history of the passions and their effects.* New York: AMS Press. (Original work published 1798)

Cuijpers, P., Berking, M., Andersson, G., Quigley, L., Kleiboer, A., & Dobson, K. S. (2013). A meta-analysis of cognitive-behavioral therapy for adult depression, alone and in comparison with other treatments. *Canadian Journal of Psychiatry, 58,* 376–385.

Diamond, A. (2005). Attention-deficit disorder (attention-deficit/hyperactivity disorder without hyperactivity): A neurobiologically and behaviorally distinct disorder from attention-deficit/hyperactivity disorder (with hyperactivity). *Development and Psychopathology, 17,* 807–825.

DuPaul, G. J., & Langberg, J. M. (2015). Educational impairments in children with ADHD. In R. A. Barkley (Ed.), *Attention-deficit hyperactivity disorder: A handbook for diagnosis and treatment* (4th ed., pp. 169–190). New York: Guilford Press.

DuPaul, J., Power, T. J., Anastopoulos, A. D., & Reid, R. (2016). *ADHD Rating Scale–5 for Children and Adolescents: Checklists, norms, and clinical interpretation.* New York: Guilford Press.

Fassbender, C., Krafft, C. E., & Schweitzer, J. B. (2015). Differentiating SCT and inattentive symptoms of ADHD using fMRI measures of cognitive control. *NeuroImage: Clinical, 8,* 390–397.

Flannery, A. J., Luebbe, A. M., & Becker, S. P. (2016). Sluggish cognitive tempo is associated with poorer study skills, more executive functioning deficits, and greater impairment in college students. *Journal of Clinical Psychology, 73*(9), 1091–1113.

Frazier, T. W., Demaree, H. A., & Youngstrom, E. A. (2004). Meta-analysis of intellectual and neuropsychological test performance in attention-deficit/hyperactivity disorder. *Neuropsychology, 18*(3), 543–555.

Froehlich, T. E., Becker, S. P., Nick, T. G., Brinkman, W. B., Stein, M. A., Peugh, J., et al. (in press). Does sluggish cognitive tempo predict methylphenidate response in a randomized controlled trial of children with ADHD? *Journal of Clinical Psychiatry.*

Garner, A. A., Hansen, A., Baxley, C., Becker, S. P., Sidol, C. A., & Beebe, D. W. (2016). Impact of sleep extension on sluggish cognitive tempo symptoms and driving behavior among adolescents with chronic short sleep. *Sleep Medicine, 30,* 93–96.

Garner, A. A., Marceaux, J. C., Mrug, S., Patterson, C., & Hodgens, B. (2010). Dimensions and correlates of attention deficit/hyperactivity disorder and sluggish cognitive tempo. *Journal of Abnormal Child Psychology, 38,* 1097–1107.

Gioia, G. A., Isquith, P. K., Guy, S. C., & Kenworthy, L. (2000). *BRIEF: Behavior Rating Inventory of Executive Function—Professional manual.* Odessa, FL: Psychological Assessment Resources.

Graham, D. M., Crocker, N., Deweese, B. N., Roesch, S. C., Coles, C. D., Kable, J. A., et al. (2013). Prenatal alcohol exposure, attention-deficit/hyperactivity disorder, and sluggish cognitive tempo. *Alcoholism: Clinical and Experimental Research, 37,* 338–346.

Harrington, K. M., & Waldman, I. D. (2010). Evaluating the utility of sluggish cognitive tempo in discriminating among DSM-IV subtypes. *Journal of Abnormal Child Psychology, 38,* 173–184.

Hartman, C. A., Willcutt, E. G., Rhee, S. H., & Pennington, B. F. (2004). The relation between sluggish cognitive tempo and DSM-IV ADHD. *Journal of Abnormal Child Psychology, 32,* 491–503.

Hervey, A. S., Epstein, J. N., & Curry, J. F. (2004). Neuropsychology of adults with attention-deficit/hyperactivity disorder: A meta-analytic review. *Neuropsychology, 18*(3), 485–503.

Hinshaw, S. P. (2002). Is ADHD an impairing condition in childhood and adolescence? In P. S. Jensen (Ed.), *Attention deficit hyperactivity disorder: State of the science—best practices.* (pp. 5-1–5-21). Kingston, NJ: Civic Research Institute.

Hoffman, H. (1865). *Der Struwwelpeter.* Erlangen, Germany: Pestalozzi-Verlag.

Huang-Pollock, C. L., Nigg, J. T., & Carr, T. H. (2005). Deficient attention is hard to find: Applying the perceptual load model of selective attention to attention deficit hyperactivity disorder subtypes. *Journal of Child Psychology and Psychiatry, 46,* 1211–1218.

Jacobson, A. L., Geist, M., & Mahone, M. (2017, February 8). Sluggish cognitive tempo, processing speed, and internalizing symptoms: The moderating effect of age. *Journal of Abnormal Child Psychology.* Epub ahead of print.

Jacobson, A. L., Murphy-Bowman, S. C., Pritchard, A. E., Tart-Zelvin, A., Zabel, T. A., & Mahone, E. M. (2012). Factor structure of a sluggish cognitive tempo scale in clinically-referred children. *Journal of Abnormal Child Psychology, 40,* 1327–1337.

Jacobson, N. S., Roberts, L. J., Berns, S. B., & McGlinchey, J. B. (1999). Methods for defining and determining the clinical significance of treatment effects: Description, application, and alternatives. *Journal of Consulting and Clinical Psychology, 67,* 300–307.

Jacobson, N. S., & Truax, P. (1991). Clinical significance: A statistical approach to defining meaningful change in psychotherapy research. *Journal of Consulting and Clinical Psychology, 59,* 12–19.

Jarrett, M. A., Rapport, H. F., Rondon, A. T., & Becker, S. P. (2014). ADHD dimensions and sluggish cognitive tempo symptoms in relation to self-report and laboratory measures of neuropsychological functioning in college students. *Journal of Attention Disorders, 21,* 673–683.

Jimenez, A. A., Ballabriga, M. C. J., Martin, A. B., Arrufat, F. J., & Giacobo, R. S. (2013). Executive functioning in children and adolescents with sluggish cognitive tempo and ADHD. *Journal of Attention Disorders, 19,* 507–514.

Khada, G., Burns, G. L., & Becker, S. P. (2016). Internal and external validity of sluggish cognitive tempo and ADHD inattention dimensions in teacher ratings of Nepali children. *Journal of Psychopathology and Behavioral Assessment, 38,* 433–442.

Koriakin, T. A., Mahone, M., & Jacobson, L. A. (2015). Sleep difficulties are associated with parent report of sluggish cognitive tempo. *Journal of Developmental and Behavioral Pediatrics, 36,* 717–723.

Lahey, B. B., Schaughency, E., Strauss, C., & Frame, C. (1984). Are attention deficit disorders with and without hyperactivity similar or dissimilar disorders? *Journal of the American Academy of Child Psychiatry, 23,* 302–309.

Langberg, J. M., Becker, S. P., & Dvorsky, M. R. (2014). The association between sluggish cognitive tempo and academic functioning in youth with attention-deficit/hyperactivity disorder (ADHD). *Journal of Abnormal Child Psychology, 42,* 91–103.

Langberg, J. M., Becker, S. P., Dvorsky, M. R., & Luebbe, A. M. (2014). Are sluggish cognitive tempo and daytime sleepiness distinct constructs? *Psychological Assessment, 26,* 586–597.

Lee, S. Y., Burns, G. L., & Becker, S. P. (2016, April 22). Toward establishing the transcultural validity of sluggish cognitive tempo: Evidence from a sample of South Korean children. *Journal of Clinical Child and Adolescent Psychology.* Epub ahead of print.

Lee, S. Y., Burns, G. L., Snell, J., & McBurnett, K. (2013). Validity of the sluggish cognitive tempo symptom dimension in children: Sluggish cognitive tempo and ADHD-inattention as distinct symptom dimensions. *Journal of Abnormal Child Psychology, 42,* 7–19.

Leikauf, J. E., & Solanto, M. V. (2016). Sluggish cognitive tempo, internalizing symptoms, and executive function in adults with ADHD. *Journal of Attention Disorders, 21*(8), 701–711.

Leopold, D. R., Christopher, M. E., Burns, G. L., Becker, S. P., Olson, R. K., & Willcutt, E. G. (2016). Attention-deficit/hyperactivity disorder and sluggish cognitive tempo throughout childhood: Temporal invariance and stability from preschool through ninth grade. *Journal of Child Psychology and Psychiatry, 57,* 1066–1074.

Lundervold, A. J., Posserud, M. B., Ullebo, A. K., Sorensen, L., & Gillberg, C. (2011). Teacher reports of hypoactivity symptoms reflect slow cognitive processing speed in primary school children. *European Child and Adolescent Psychiatry, 20,* 121–126.

Markovich-Pilon, A. N., Corkum, P. V., & Joyce, A. M. (2017). Sluggish cognitive tempo: Investigating associated daytime and nighttime impairments. *The ADHD Report, 25*(3), 1–5.

Marshall, S. A., Evans, S. W., Eiraldi, R. B., Becker, S. P., & Power, T. J. (2013). Social and academic impairment in youth with ADHD, predominantly inattentive type and sluggish cognitive tempo. *Journal of Abnormal Child Psychology, 42,* 77–90.

Mash, E. J., & Barkley, R. A. (Eds.). (2003). *Child psychopathology.* New York: Guilford Press.

Maurer, R. G., & Stewart, M. (1980). Attention deficit disorder without hyperactivity in a child psychiatric clinic. *Journal of Clinical Psychiatry, 41,* 232–233.

McBurnett, K., Clemow, D., Williams, D., Villodas, M., Wietecha, L., & Barkley, R. (2017). Atomoxetine-related change in sluggish cognitive tempo is partially independent of change in attention-deficit/hyperactivity disorder inattentive symptoms. *Journal of Child and Adolescent Psychopharmacology, 27,* 38–42.

McBurnett, K., Pfiffner, L. J., & Frick, P. J. (2001). Symptom properties as a function of

ADHD type: An argument for continued study of sluggish cognitive tempo. *Journal of Abnormal Child Psychology, 29,* 207–213.

McBurnett, K., Villodas, M., Burns, G. L., Hinshaw, S. P., Beaulieu, A., & Pfiffner, L. J. (2014). Structure and validity of sluggish cognitive tempo using an expanded item pool in children with attention-deficit/hyperactivity disorder. *Journal of Abnormal Child Psychology, 42,* 37–48.

McConaughy, S. H., & Achenbach, T. M. (2001). *Child Behavior Checklist—Direct Observation Form.* Burlington, VT: Authors.

McConaughy, S. H., Ivanova, M., Antshel, K., & Eiraldi, R. B. (2009). Standardized observational assessment of attention deficit/hyperactivity disorder combined and predominantly inattentive subtypes: I. Test session observations. *School Psychology Review, 38,* 45–66.

McConaughy, S. H., Ivanova, M., Antshel, K., Eiraldi, R. B., & Dumenci, L. (2009). Standardized observational assessment of attention deficit/hyperactivity disorder combined and predominantly inattentive subtypes: II. Classroom observations. *School Psychology Review, 39,* 362–381.

McGrath, L. M., Hutaff-Lee, C., Scott, A., Boada, R., Shriberg, L. D., & Pennington, B. F. (2008). Children with comorbid speech sound disorder and specific language impairment are at increased risk for attention-deficit/hyperactivity disorder. *Journal of Abnormal Child Psychology, 36,* 151–163.

McQuade, J. D., & Hoza, B. (2015). Peer relationships of children with ADHD. In R. A. Barkley (Ed.), *Attention-deficit hyperactivity disorder: A handbook for diagnosis and treatment* (4th ed., pp. 210–222). New York: Guilford Press.

Mikami, A. Y., Huang-Pollack, C. L., Pfiffner, L. J., McBurnett, K., & Hangai, D. (2007). Social skills differences among attention-deficit/hyperactivity disorder types in a chat room assessment task. *Journal of Abnormal Child Psychology, 35,* 509–521.

Milich, R., Ballentine, A. C., & Lynam, D. R. (2001). ADHD/combined type and ADHD/predominantly inattentive type are distinct and unrelated disorders. *Clinical Psychology: Science and Practice, 8,* 463–488.

Mirsky, A. F. (1996). Disorders of attention. In R. G. Lyon & N. A. Krasnegor (Eds.), *Attention, memory, and executive function* (pp. 71–96). Baltimore: Brookes.

Mitchell, J. T., Knouse, L. E., Nelson-Gray, R. O., & Kwapil, T. R. (2009). Self-reported ADHD symptoms among college students: Item position affects symptom endorsement rates. *Journal of Attention Disorders, 13,* 154–160.

Moruzzi, S., Rijsdijk, F., & Battaglia, M. (2014). A twin study of the relationships among inattention, hyperactivity–impulsivity and sluggish cognitive tempo problems. *Journal of Abnormal Child Psychology, 42,* 63–75.

Mueller, A. K., Tucha, L., Koerts, J., Groen, Y., Lange, K. W., & Tucha, O. (2014). Sluggish cognitive tempo and its neurocognitive, social, and emotional correlates: A systematic review of the current literature. *Journal of Molecular Psychiatry, 2*(1), 5.

Olfson, M., Marcus, S. C., Weissman, M. M., & Jensen, P. S. (2002). National trends in the use of psychotropic medications by children. *Journal of the American Academy of Child and Adolescent Psychiatry, 41,* 514–521.

Palmer, E. D., & Finger, S. (2001). An early description of ADHD (inattentive subtype): Dr. Alexander Crichton and "mental restlessness" (1798). *Child Psychology and Psychiatry Review, 6,* 66–73.

Penny, A. M., Waschbusch, D. A., Klein, R. M., Corkum, P., & Eskes, G. (2009). Developing a measure of sluggish cognitive tempo for children: Content validity, factor structure, and reliability. *Psychological Assessment, 21,* 380–389.

Pfiffner, L. J., Mikami, A. Y., Huang-Pollock, C., Easterlin, B., Zalecki, C., & McBurnett, K. (2007). A randomized, controlled trial of integrated home–school behavioral treatment for ADHD, predominantly inattentive type. *Journal of the American Academy of Child and Adolescent Psychiatry, 48,* 1041–1050.

Pliszka, S. (2015). Comorbid psychiatric disorders in children with ADHD. In R. A. Barkley (Ed.), *Attention-deficit hyperactivity disorder: A handbook for diagnosis and treatment* (4th ed., pp. 140–168). New York: Guilford Press.

Preszler, J., Burns, G. L., Litson, K., Geiser, C., Servera, M., & Becker, S. P. (2017, January 1). How consistent is sluggish cognitive tempo across occasions, sources, and settings?: Evidence from latent state–trait modeling. *Assessment.* Epub ahead of print.

Raiker, J. S., Greening, L., Stoppelbein, L., Becker, S. P., Fite, P. J., & Luebbe, A. M. (2015). Mediating effect of psychopathy on the risk of social problems among children with ADHD versus sluggish cognitive tempo symptoms. *Child Psychiatry and Human Development, 46,* 523–532.

Reeves, C. B., Palmer, S., Gross, A. M., Simonian, S. J., Taylor, L., Willigham, E., et al. (2007). Brief report: Sluggish cognitive tempo among pediatric survivors of acute lymphoblastic leukemia. *Journal of Pediatric Psychology, 32,* 1050–1054.

Reynolds, C., & Kamphaus, R. (2004). *Behavior Assessment System for Children–II.* Circle Pines, MN: American Guidance Service.

Roberts, R. E., Attkisson, C. C., & Rosenblatt, A. (1998). Prevalence of psychopathology among children and adolescents. *American Journal of Psychiatry, 155,* 715–725.

Rowe, R., Maughan, B., & Goodman, R. (2004). Childhood psychiatric disorder and unintentional injury: Findings from a national cohort study. *Journal of Pediatric Psychology, 29,* 119–130.

Saxbe, C., & Barkley, R. A. (2014). The other attention disorder?: Sluggish cognitive tempo vs. ADHD—update for clinicians. *Journal of Clinical Psychiatry, 20,* 38–49.

Servera, M., Bernad, M., Carillo, J. M., Collado, S., & Burns, G. L. (2016). Longitudinal correlates of sluggish cognitive tempo and ADHD-inattention symptom dimensions with Spanish children. *Journal of Clinical Child and Adolescent Psychology, 45,* 632–641.

Shelton, C. R., Addison, W. E., & Hartung, C. M. (2017). ADHD and SCT symptomatology in relation to college students' use of self-regulated learning strategies. *Journal of Attention Disorders.* Epub ahead of print.

Skirbekk, B., Hansen, B. H., Oerbeck, B., & Kristensen, H. (2011). The relationship between sluggish cognitive tempo, subjects of attention-deficit/hyperactivity disorder, and anxiety disorders. *Journal of Abnormal Child Psychology, 39,* 513–525.

Smallwood, J., Fishman, D., & Schooler, J. (2007). Counting the cost of an absent mind: Mind wandering as an under recognized influence on educational performance. *Psychonomic Bulletin and Review, 14,* 230–236.

Smallwood, J., & Schooler, J. (2006). The restless mind. *Psychological Bulletin, 132,* 946–958.

Smith, Z. R., & Langberg, J. M. (2017, May 19). Predicting academic impairment and internalizing psychopathology using a multidimensional framework of sluggish cognitive tempo with parent- and adolescent reports. *European Child and Adolescent Psychiatry, 26*(9), 1141–1150.

Tamm, L., Brenner, S. B., Bamberger, M. E., & Becker, S. P. (2018). Are sluggish cognitive tempo symptoms associated with executive functioning in preschoolers? *Child Neuropsychology, 24*(1), 82–105.

Tamm, L., Garner, A. A., Loren, R. E. A., Epstein, J. N., Vaughn, A. J., Ciesielski, H. A., et al. (2016). Slow sluggish cognitive tempo symptoms are associated with poorer academic performance in children with ADHD. *Psychiatry Research, 242,* 251–259.

Thomas, C. P., Conrad, P., Casler, R., & Goodman, E. (2006). Trends in the use of psychotropic medications among adolescents, 1994–2001. *Psychiatric Services, 57,* 63–69.

Thorell, L. B., & Nyberg, L. (2008). The Childhood Executive Functioning Inventory

(CHEXI): A new rating instrument for parents and teachers. *Developmental Neuropsychology, 33,* 536–552.

Todd, R. D., Rasmussen, E. R., Wood, C., Levy, F., & Hay, D. (2004). Should sluggish cognitive tempo symptoms be included in the diagnosis of attention-deficit/hyperactivity disorder? *Journal of the American Academy of Child and Adolescent Psychiatry, 43,* 588–597.

Toplak, M. E., West, R. F., & Stanovich, K. E. (2013). Practitioner review: Do performance-based measures and ratings of executive function assess the same construct? *Journal of Child Psychology and Psychiatry, 54,* 113–224.

Wahlstedt, C., & Bohlin, G. (2010). DSM-IV defined inattention and sluggish cognitive tempo: Independent and interactive relations to neuropsychological factors and comorbidity. *Child Neuropsychology, 16*(4), 250–365.

Watabe, Y., Owens, J. S., Evans, S. W., & Brandt, N. E. (2013). The relationship between sluggish cognitive tempo and impairment in children with and without ADHD. *Journal of Abnormal Child Psychology, 42,* 105–115.

Weinberg, W. A., & Brumback, R. A. (1990). Primary disorder of vigilance: A novel explanation of inattentiveness, daydreaming, boredom, restlessness, and sleepiness. *Journal of Pediatrics, 116,* 720–725.

Weinberg, W. A., & Brumback, R. A. (1992). The myth of attention deficit-hyperactivity disorder: Symptoms resulting from multiple causes. *Journal of Child Neurology, 7,* 431–445.

Weinberg, W. A., & Harper, C. R. (1993). Vigilance and its disorders. *Neurology Clinics, 11,* 59–78.

Wietecha, L., Williams, D., Shaywitz, S., Shaywitz, B., Hooper, S. R., Wigal, S. B., et al. (2013). Atomoxetine improved attention in children and adolescents with attention-deficit/hyperactivity disorder and dyslexia in a 16 week, acute, randomized, double-blind trial. *Journal of Child and Adolescent Psychopharmacology, 23,* 605–609.

Willcutt, E. G. (2015). Theories of ADHD. In R. A. Barkley (Ed.), *Attention-deficit hyperactivity disorder: A handbook for diagnosis and treatment* (3rd ed., pp. 391–404). New York: Guilford Press.

Willcutt, E. G., Chhabildas, N., Kinnear, M., DeFries, J. C., Olson, R. K., Leopold, D. R., et al. (2013). The internal and external validity of sluggish cognitive tempo and its relation with DSM-IV ADHD. *Journal of Abnormal Child Psychology, 42,* 21–35.

Willcutt, E. G., Doyle, A. E., Nigg, J. T., Faraone, S. V., & Pennington, B. F. (2005). Validity of the executive function theory of attention-deficit/hyperactivity disorder: A meta-analytic review. *Biological Psychiatry, 57,* 1336–1346.

Willcutt, E. G., Nigg, E. T., Pennington, B. F., Solanto, M. V., Rohde, L. A., Tannock, R., et al. (2012). Validity of the DSM-IV attention deficit/hyperactivity disorder symptom dimensions and subtypes. *Journal of Abnormal Psychology, 121,* 991–1010.

Wood, W. L. M., Lewandowski, L. J., Lovett, B. J., & Antshel, K. M. (2017). Executive dysfunction and functional impairment associated with sluggish cognitive tempo in emerging adulthood. *Journal of Attention Disorders, 21,* 691–700.

Wood, W. L. M., Potts, H. E., Lewandowski, L. J., & Lovett, B. J. (2016). Sluggish cognitive tempo and speed of performance. *Journal of Attention Disorders, 21,* 684–690.

Zito, J. M., Safer, D. J., dosReis, S., Gardner, J. F., Magder, L., Soeken, K., et al. (2003). Psychotropic practice patterns for youth: A 10-year perspective. *Archives of Pediatric and Adolescent Medicine, 157,* 17–25.

Index

Note. *f* or *t* following a page number indicates a figure or a table.